Penile Color Duplex-Doppler Ultrasound in Erectile Dysfunction Diagnosis and Management

Eduardo de Paula Miranda • Felipe Carneiro

Penile Color Duplex-Doppler Ultrasound in Erectile Dysfunction Diagnosis and Management

A Complete Guide to Best Practices

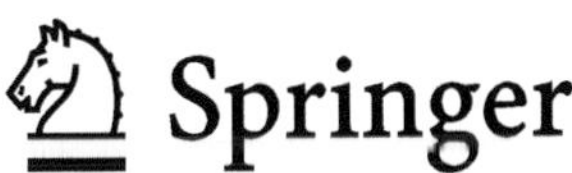

Springer

Eduardo de Paula Miranda
Centro Universitário Christus
(UNICHRISTUS)
Fortaleza, Ceará, Brazil

Felipe Carneiro
Radiology Department
University of São Paulo
São Paulo, São Paulo, Brazil

ISBN 978-3-031-55651-7   ISBN 978-3-031-55649-4   (eBook)
https://doi.org/10.1007/978-3-031-55649-4

This Springer imprint is published by the registered company Springer Nature Switzerland AG
The registered company address is: Gewerbestrasse 11, 6330 Cham, Switzerland

Paper in this product is recyclable.

Preface

It is with great satisfaction that we present this comprehensive and innovative guide on Doppler ultrasound of the penis with pharmacologically induced erections for the evaluation of erectile dysfunction and penile deformities. This is the result of the hard work and passionate dedication of two dedicated Brazilian authors. This book represents the fruit of a friendship and partnership developed around the deepest desire to standardize and disseminate this diagnostic tool, which has long suffered from the skepticism of the medical community due to the inconsistency of its results.

These authors demonstrate tireless dedication to the method and its technical refinement and have undertaken a colossal task: to create the best guide to penile Doppler ever conceived. After years of research experience and training hundreds of physicians in this methodology, they have gathered and synthesized the vast knowledge available in international medical literature and adapted it to the current reality of medical practice. Moreover, they have committed to a high-quality standardization system that helps physicians develop consistency in conducting the examination and its interpretation, always based on the honesty and integrity that permeate every page of this guide.

The importance of diagnosing and treating erectile dysfunction and penile deformities cannot be underestimated. These conditions affect not only physical health but also the quality of life and self-esteem of patients. Until recently, penile Doppler ultrasound was an underutilized and underestimated tool for assessing these conditions. However, the authors of this book understand that the incorporation of this advanced technique can revolutionize how we approach men's health issues.

This book is divided into 17 carefully organized chapters, each addressing specific aspects of penile Doppler ultrasound. From basic anatomy to the most complex clinical cases, the authors provide a gradual and didactic approach that serves both beginners and experienced professionals in the fields of Urology, Radiology, and Sexual Medicine. The text is complemented by high-quality images that accurately illustrate the suggested procedures.

One of the most remarkable aspects of this guide is the practical and standardized approach proposed by the authors. In a medical field that often lacks clear protocols and specific guidelines, this technical material provides a detailed, step-by-step roadmap for conducting examinations, interpreting results, and making evidence-based clinical decisions. Additionally, the authors acknowledge the method's limitations and suggest possible approaches to inconclusive results. This not only simplifies the work of healthcare professionals but also ensures quality and consistent patient care.

In addition to the technical approach, this guide also emphasizes the importance of ethics in medical practice, as penile Doppler is highly operator-dependent. Unethical examiners can have disastrous consequences for both patients and credibility of the method. The authors recognize that while medicine is an ever-evolving science full of relative truths, honesty and patient well-being must always come first. Readers are encouraged to always adopt an ethical perspective and a critical approach in daily practice.

We hope that as readers progress through the pages of this book, they will absorb the depth of knowledge and the commitment to excellence demonstrated by the authors. It is our hope that this guide becomes an invaluable reference for physicians, medical students, and all healthcare professionals involved in the diagnosis and treatment of sexual dysfunctions. Moreover, we hope this book inspires a new generation of practitioners to adopt high standards of clinical practice and contribute to the advancement of sexual medicine globally.

In conclusion, we enthusiastically recommend this book to readers. It not only represents the state of the art in penile Doppler ultrasound but also incorporates the fundamental values that should guide medical practice. This humble work aspires to be the best guide ever created on the subject and a testament to the authors' commitment to the health and well-being of their patients.

<table>
<tr><td>Fortaleza, Ceará, Brazil</td><td>Eduardo de Paula Miranda</td></tr>
<tr><td>São Paulo, São Paulo, Brazil</td><td>Felipe Carneiro</td></tr>
</table>

Contents

Chapter 1
History of Functional Assessment of Penile Erection

1.1   Introduction

Sexual health is considered a key aspect of overall health since it has a substantial impact on quality of life, and an increasing interest in this subject has been currently being observed. Even if it is naturally expected that a man's sexuality might deteriorate with aging, most men consider sexual activity important throughout maturity and into extremely elder years. In a recent global study of sexuality among persons between the ages of 40 and 80, 82% of males agreed with the statement that satisfying sex is vital to maintain a relationship, and 80% of men said they had sexual contact at least once in the year prior to the interview [1]. Additionally, since the majority of men who present with ED do not only participate in solitary sexual activity, partner satisfaction is another crucial factor for determining sexual satisfaction [1]. ED is defined by the National Institutes of Health (NIH) Consensus Panel as the inability to achieve and/or sustain a penile erection sufficient for fulfilling sexual activity [2]. According to studies in the late 1990s, more than 25 million men aged 40–70 years had ED in the United States and around 150 million men worldwide [3], and these number are increasing exponentially with the aging population with estimates that we have already reached over 300 million men around the globe [4–6].

Regardless of the underlying reason of ED, the loss of penile rigidity is considered one of the most unpleasant situations for most men. ED can have a severe negative impact on their psychological health, as a healthy erection is very important to the sense of masculinity. Moreover, men usually feel uncomfortable discussing their concerns about erection issues with their sexual partner since they may view it as a humiliating issue and try to hide it [7]. The subsequent behavioral adjustments such as refraining from any physical contact or greater levels of intimacy with their partner are likely to have a negative impact on the relationship as a whole, which will

E. d. P. Miranda, F. Carneiro, *Penile Color Duplex-Doppler Ultrasound in
Erectile Dysfunction Diagnosis and Management*,
https://doi.org/10.1007/978-3-031-55649-4_1

exacerbate their feeling of social exclusion and increase their psychological suffering. In men with ED, depressive symptoms are frequent and occasionally severe enough to fulfill the criteria for major depressive disorder [8], and contribute significantly to relationship issues, as reports have shown that more than 20% of men with ED claimed that their relationship had terminated as a direct result of their erection problem [7].

Many techniques have been described in sexual medicine history to assess penile erection in the ED context. Some diagnostic methods are noninvasive, while others are invasive. The development of phosphodiesterase type 5 inhibitors for the treatment of ED was a turning point as many clinicians began to handle the majority of ED cases in a goal-oriented rather than a cause-oriented manner. So, further diagnostic testing by a specialist may be necessary depending on the nature of the issue and the patient's interest, particularly when these drugs are contraindicated or fail to treat ED [8].

1.2 Noninvasive Methods to Penile Erection Assessment

1.2.1 Nocturnal Penile Tumescence and Rigidity Tests

Nocturnal penile tumescence and rigidity (NPTR) testing can assist distinguishing between organic and psychogenic ED and give the patient an accurate assessment of his capacity for an erection. This test is usually performed using tools such as RigiScan (Fig. 1.1), mercury strain gauges, or simple straps that are adjusted around the penis in order to be able to capture and eventually measure nocturnal tumescence. Due to the noninvasive nature of RigiScan, it used to be very popular. Some limitations of NPTR testing are that some patients with psychogenic ED and sleep disturbances might also have abnormal results and that it was not able to identify some alterations in axial penile rigidity. It is a known fact that the best physical indicator of an erect penis' ability to resist vaginal compressive forces during pelvic thrusting and vaginal intromission is axial stiffness [9].

1.2.2 Visual Sexual Stimulation Plethysmography (VSS)

Diurnal penile plethysmography for evaluation of erection during visual sexual stimuli has a significant historical value since it was the first reported way to employ pornography, either erotic movies or photographs, to evaluate sexual arousal in ED patients. It was another technique to distinguish between organic and psychogenic ED causes. VSS was helpful for researchers who were willing to assess the quality of an erection or to perform an in-office evaluation of penile deformities such as congenital curvatures or Peyronie's disease. Some patients would also benefit from

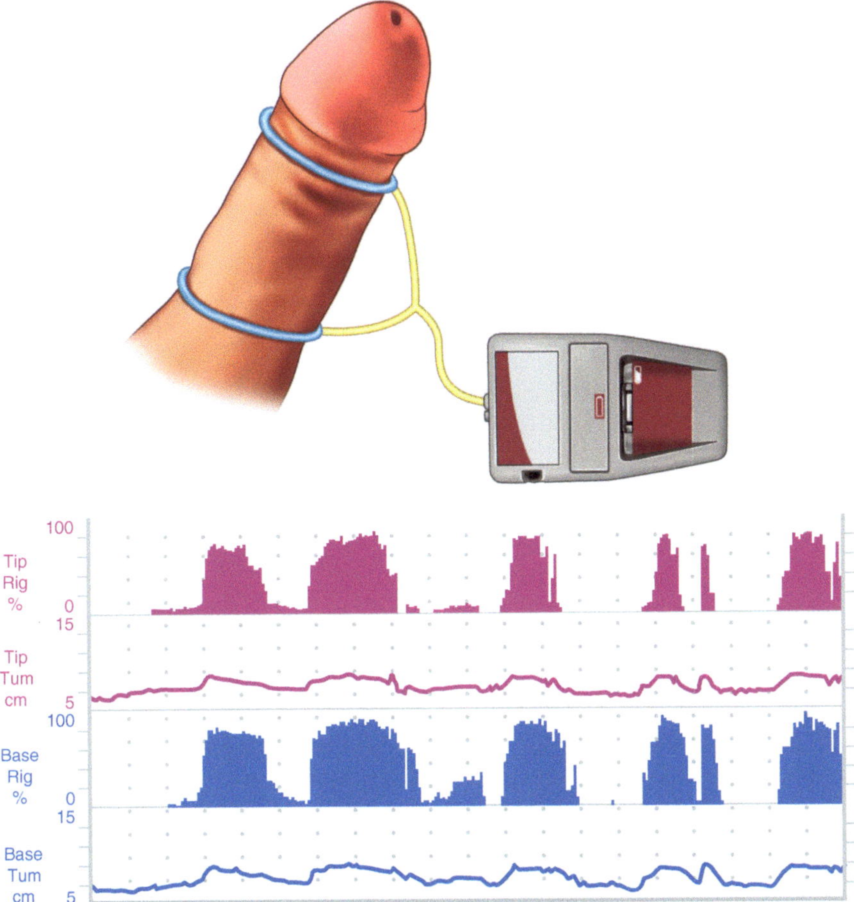

Fig. 1.1 RigiScan device with nocturnal readings of pressure increasing pressure in both rings consistent of physiological nocturnal erections

a more objective self-evaluation of the erection's quality objectively, which could aid in regaining self-confidence. When the NPTR test was negative, a positive VSS was interesting, especially if the patient was unable to fall asleep in the lab [10].

1.2.3   Questionnaires

Questionnaires for patient self-report outcomes have become the gold standard for evaluating male sexual function since the late 1990s, as they became very popular during PDE5i trials. Overall, they are considered simple-to-use clinical tools for the detection of ED that could be routinely used in clinical practice. There are many available psychometric instruments in form of questionnaires that have been validated. However, the International Index of Erectile Function (IIEF) is perhaps the most widely accepted for such purpose. It is a psychometrically valid and reliable tool with 15 items and 5 domains of male sexual function and was created in cooperation with a global panel of specialists to assess the efficacy of treatment in controlled clinical studies [11]. The IIEF offers good sensitivity and specificity for identifying actual therapeutic effects in men with ED regardless of etiology. Later on, an abridged version of the IIEF was created, reducing the number of questions from 15 to 5 in order to provide an abbreviated version to evaluate erectile function more specifically [12]. Four of the five questions in this condensed version pertain to erection quality. It is important to highlight that in spite of being useful for the diagnosis and severity classification of ED, the IIEF-5 does not necessarily indicate organicity. A more detailed discussion regarding the use of IIEF in the evaluation of penile rigidity is provided in Chap. 8.

1.2.4   Hormonal Tests

It is a well-known fact that testosterone affects many aspects of the male sexual function, most notably sexual desire. Though not fully understood, there has also been accumulating evidence that low testosterone levels have a negative effect on the normal physiology of erection. According to classic research, 10–20% of men with ED and up to 35% of men over 60 have hormonal deficiency [13]. It is now known that human sexual desire and erectile function both respond to androgens, but at possibly distinct threshold levels. The capacity of the penile smooth muscle and endothelial cells to relax may be diminished as a result of varying degrees of testosterone deprivation, without significantly influencing sexual desire. Additionally, the expression and activity of phosphodiesterase type-5 in the human corpus cavernosum may be directly regulated by androgens [13]. Therefore, evaluation of a full hormonal panel including testosterone levels is usually recommended for men with ED, although it does not constitute a direct measure of a man's sexual/erectile function.

1.3   Invasive Methods for Penile Erection Assessment

1.3.1   Angiography and Dynamic Infusion Cavernosography/ Cavernosometry

The gold standard for identifying arterial anomalies is selective penile arteriography. The internal iliac artery, which gives rise to the internal pudendal artery, which in turn provides the common penile artery, and finally the cavernosal artery, is the most common source of blood supply for the corpus cavernosum [14]. Evaluation of the penile, cavernosal, and dorsal arteries on either side is made possible by intra-corporal injection of papaverine, followed by selective injection of the pudendal artery with contrast material. It is possible to identify arterial stenoses and occlusions. However, this is an invasive procedure that is expensive and time-consuming and may be painful.

On the other hand, the ultimate diagnosis of corporal veno-occlusive disorder (CVOD) is ideally given using dynamic infusion cavernosometry and cavernosography (DICC). This technique involves the insertion of two butterfly needles, one in each corporal body, with one connected to a pressure transducer and the other to a servo-controlled pump. Upon the administration of vasoactive agents, an erection is induced and several parameters can be measured. The first phase involves assessing the development of intracavernosal pressure (ICP) within the corpus cavernosum (measured in mmHg). Secondly, the examiners should measure veno-occlusive function by determining flow-to-maintain values, which refers to the flow of saline in mL/min required to sustain a given ICP defined by the pump, and pressure decay assessment, which measures the pressure drop from a starting ICP of 150 mmHg over 30 s (measured in mmHg/30 s). The last phase involves determining cavernosal artery inflow gradients measured in mmHg, which refers to the difference between brachial artery systolic pressure and the cavernosal artery occlusion pressure [15]. The cavernosography phase is considered optional by some authors and is performed with a flush injection of contrast media to allow for an anatomic evaluation of the cavernous bodies. Some of the potential drawbacks of DICC are its invasive nature, the prolonged duration required to conduct the procedure, and the absence of standardized criteria for defining venous leak and arterial insufficiency during the assessment.

Arteriography and DICC are considered more invasive diagnostic methods and are very rarely performed nowadays. Their use has been reserved for very selected cases, especially for those with persistent abnormal penile Doppler ultrasound and who are possible candidates for vascular reconstructive surgery [15].

1.3.2   Intracavernous Injection Test (IIT)

An in-office intracavernous injection test is a frequently used screening method in the clinical evaluation of individuals with ED. Following the intracavernous delivery of vasoactive drugs either with or without additional manual, vibratory, or audiovisual sexual stimulation, an erectile response is usually expected. The test is rather straightforward, minimally invasive, and almost painless, and may be performed without the need of any additional monitoring device. A normal erectile response is considered when a rigid and sustained erection is observed. The erectile response is thought to ultimately reflect the hemodynamic status of the erectile mechanism, which is the basis of the IIT's diagnostic component. It has been suggested that a positive erectile response is accurate enough to rule out serious venous leak and arterial insufficiency, but not neurogenic or psychogenic ED. However, there are insufficient hemodynamic data to support the diagnostic accuracy of a positive IIT response. In fact, intracavernous injection experiments performed on individuals with known hemodynamic impairment have shown positive results as well [14].

1.3.3   Penile Doppler Ultrasound with Intracavernous Injection (PDU)

In 1985, Lue et al. combined for the first time the intracavernous injection of a vasoactive agent and penile Doppler ultrasound (PDU) to assess penile hemodynamics, describing a diagnostic modality to identify arterial insufficiency and CVOD in patients with ED in a less invasive fashion. Since PDU's first introduction, IIT has been largely replaced by PDU because IIT yields limited diagnostic information regarding vascular status, and it is often considered inconclusive as a diagnostic procedure. The added information from the PDU may provide a clear diagnosis and allow for targeted treatment, which could increase treatment efficacy and patient satisfaction [16].

1.4   Conclusion

Currently, PDU is the method of choice for assessing penile hemodynamics of men with ED. PDU is significantly less invasive and more accessible than other classic penile hemodynamics studies such as angiography and cavernosography/cavernosometry. Peak systolic velocity (PSV) value allows for direct evaluation of the arterial supply, and end-diastolic velocity (EDV) provides an indirect evaluation of the veno-occlusive mechanism. However, maximum smooth muscle relaxation is required in both erectile tissue and cavernous arteries for this approach to produce reliable and reproducible results. A mistaken diagnosis of arterial insufficiency and/ or CVOD may result from excessive sympathetic discharge, as it inhibits complete smooth muscle relaxation in response to vasoactive drugs. Several tactics, including redosing schedules of vasoactive agents and audiovisual sexual stimulation, have been proposed to prevent incorrect diagnosis during PDU. All different nuances of PDU will be discussed in subsequent chapters, including protocols, problems, and a strategy for writing a comprehensive report, as it is the main purpose of this book.

References

1. Nicolosi A, Laumann EO, Glasser DB, Moreira ED Jr, Paik A, Gingell C. Sexual behavior and sexual dysfunctions after age 40: the global study of sexual attitudes and behaviors. Urology. 2004;64(5):991–7.
2. Health NIO. NIH Consensus Conference. Impotence. NIH consensus development panel on impotence. JAMA. 1993;270:83–90.

3. Laumann EO, Paik A, Rosen RC. Sexual dysfunction in the United States: prevalence and predictors. JAMA. 1999;281(6):537–44.
4. Aytaç IA, Araujo AB, Johannes CB, Kleinman KP, McKinlay JB. Socioeconomic factors and incidence of erectile dysfunction: findings of the longitudinal Massachusetts male aging study. Soc Sci Med. 2000;51(5):771–8.
5. Feldman HA, Goldstein I, Hatzichristou DG, Krane RJ, McKinlay JB. Impotence and its medical and psychosocial correlates: results of the Massachusetts male aging study. J Urol. 1994;151(1):54–61.
6. Mak R, De Backer G, Kornitzer M, De Meyer JM. Prevalence and correlates of erectile dysfunction in a population-based study in Belgium. Eur Urol. 2002;41(2):132–8.
7. Tomlinson J, Wright D. Impact of erectile dysfunction and its subsequent treatment with sildenafil: qualitative study. BMJ. 2004;328(7447):1037.
8. Fisher WA, Rosen RC, Eardley I, Niederberger C, Nadel A, Kaufman J, et al. The multinational men's attitudes to life events and sexuality (MALES) study phase II: understanding PDE5 inhibitor treatment seeking patterns, among men with erectile dysfunction. J Sex Med. 2004;1(2):150–60.
9. Yang CC, Porter MP, Penson DF. Comparison of the international index of erectile function erectile domain scores and nocturnal penile tumescence and rigidity measurements: does one predict the other? BJU Int. 2006;98(1):105–9.
10. Opsomer R-J, Wese F-X, Van Cangh P. Visual sexual stimulation plethysmography: complementary test to nocturnal penile plethysmography. Urology. 1990;35(6):504–7.
11. Rhoden E, Telöken C, Sogari P, Vargas SC. The use of the simplified international index of erectile function (IIEF-5) as a diagnostic tool to study the prevalence of erectile dysfunction. Int J Impot Res. 2002;14(4):245–50.
12. Rosen RC, Cappelleri JC, Gendrano N 3rd. The international index of erectile function (IIEF): a state-of-the-science review. Int J Impot Res. 2002;14(4):226–44.
13. Aversa A, Isidori A, De Martino M, Caprio M, Fabbrini E, Rocchietti-March M, et al. Androgens and penile erection: evidence for a direct relationship between free testosterone and cavernous vasodilation in men with erectile dysfunction. Clin Endocrinol. 2000;53(4):517–22.
14. Ma M, Yu B, Qin F, Yuan J. Current approaches to the diagnosis of vascular erectile dysfunction. Transl Androl Urol. 2020;9(2):709.
15. Levine LA. Diagnosis and treatment of erectile dysfunction. Am J Med. 2000;109(9):3–12.
16. Carneiro F, Nascimento B, Miranda EP, Cury J, Cerri GG, Chammas MC. Audiovisual sexual stimulation improves diagnostic accuracy of penile Doppler ultrasound in patients with erectile dysfunction. J Sex Med. 2020;17(2):249–56.

Chapter 2
Principles of Doppler Ultrasound

2.1 Introduction

The knowledge of the physical principles and basic concepts about diagnostic ultrasound is mandatory to understand the interaction of the sound waves with tissues, imaging formation, and, consequently, advantages, disadvantages, clinical applications, and limitations of the method.

2.2 Ultrasound Physics

A mechanical wave called sound disrupts a medium and moves energy from one place to another. The energy of the sound wave is transmitted through collisions with nearby particles as it moves through a medium. These particles oscillate around their resting positions with no net displacement. Sound waves can either be longitudinal or transverse, depending on the direction of their oscillations in relation to the direction of the energy travelling through the medium. Only solids can transmit sound waves transversely, whereas all materials can support a longitudinal wave, which is how ultrasound is transmitted through the body's soft tissues and fluid [1], which is illustrated in Fig. 2.1.

The number of oscillations (or cycles) per second is the frequency of a sound wave, which is expressed in hertz, or Hz. A particle has a frequency of 1 Hz if it oscillates fully once every second. The term "ultrasound" refers to sound waves with frequencies above 20 kilohertz (kHz), which are too high for the human ear to hear. However, the frequencies utilized in medical imaging are much higher, often 2–20 megahertz (MHz).

The length of a sound wave is the distance it travels in one cycle. It is inversely correlated with frequency, meaning that the greater the frequency, the shorter the

© The Author(s), under exclusive license to Springer Nature
Switzerland AG 2024
E. d. P. Miranda, F. Carneiro, *Penile Color Duplex-Doppler Ultrasound in
Erectile Dysfunction Diagnosis and Management*,
https://doi.org/10.1007/978-3-031-55649-4_2

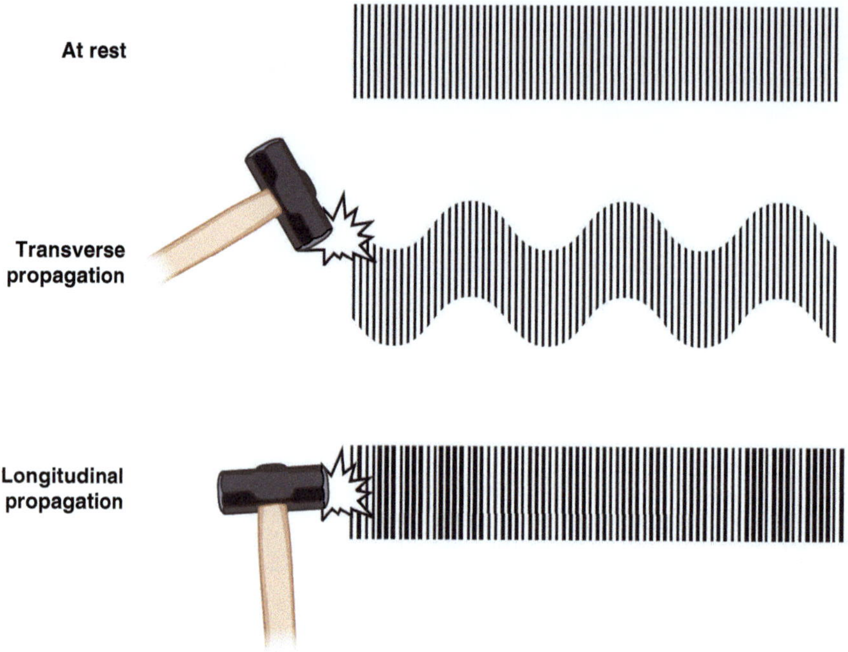

Fig. 2.1 Longitudinal propagation of a mechanical force, which happens with sound in the human tissues, or the transverse propagation of a mechanical force, which can only happen in solids

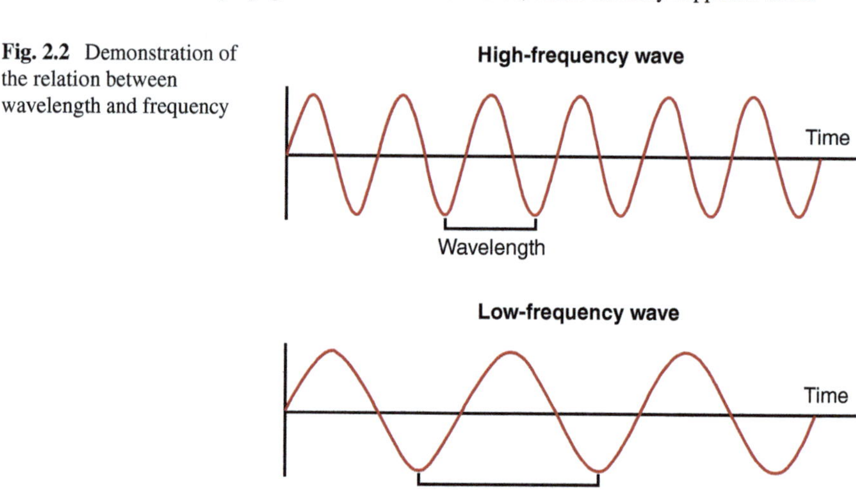

Fig. 2.2 Demonstration of the relation between wavelength and frequency

wavelength (Fig. 2.2). Images with increased resolution are produced by shorter wavelengths, but fewer soft tissues are penetrated. To generate images of deeper structures, such as the abdominal and pelvic organs, lower frequency probes are employed (2–5 MHz). On the other hand, higher frequency probes (5–20 MHz) are utilized for superficial structures, such as the visualization of peripheral vessels in the penis [1].

2.3   Creation of Ultrasound Images

An electrical current is temporarily passed through a piezoelectric crystal inside the ultrasound probe to create sound waves that will be received by the tissues. The crystal then holds off on sending the next pulse until it has received the rebounding echoes. Typically, a 1-microsecond (μs) pulse is repeated at 1-millisecond (ms) intervals. Therefore, each crystal receives the returning echoes 99.9% of the time and produces ultrasonic waves only 0.1% of the time. In fact the probe is made up of a phased array of many piezoelectric crystals that are successively triggered by electronic pulses that sweep across the probe's surface [2].

The ultrasonic wave comes into contact with interfaces between various tissues as it travels through the patient. A portion of the wave's energy is reflected and the rest is transmitted at these contacts. Some of the reflected echoes will return to the transducer if the angle between the interface and transducer is higher than 60°. The reflected sound waves are transformed into electrical pulses by the piezoelectric crystal, and these electrical pulses are then translated into a two-dimensional (2D) image. The more the energy is reflected, the brighter (or whiter) the image appears.

The differential in acoustic impedance (Z) between two tissues affects how much energy is reflected at that interface. A tissue's acoustic impedance is a function of its density and the speed at which sound waves move through it. Water and soft tissues have far greater densities than air, which in turn have much lower densities than bone. The amount of energy reflected and the brightness of the generated image increase with the size of the acoustic impedance mismatch between two materials at a contact. Less than 1% of the wave's energy is reflected when tissues with similar densities, such the liver and kidney, come together. However, almost all of the wave's energy is reflected at the boundary between soft tissue and air or bone. Since no energy is being communicated, it is impossible to learn anything about the tissues beneath this point. This explains why ultrasound is typically ineffective for evaluating the colon, lung, or inside the bone. It also describes the necessity for a coupling gel between the probe and the patient's skin and the need to prevent air bubbles to reduce reflection at the skin/probe contact [2].

Calculating the depth (d) of the tissue interface is necessary to produce a 2D picture. Through soft tissue, ultrasound moves at a constant average speed (c) of 1540 ms^{-1}. The amount of time (t) required for the ultrasonic pulse to reach the interface's distance (d) and for the reflected wave to return to the transducer is as follows:

$$t = 2d \, / \, c.$$

The tissue interface depth is, then, rearranged as follows:

$$d = ct / 2.$$

2.3.1 Sound Attenuation and Compensation

A process known as attenuation occurs as a sound wave gradually loses energy as it travels through the body. Reflection, refraction, scatter, and absorption are the causes of this phenomenon (Fig. 2.3). Refraction and reflection take place where tissues meet. The creation of the necessary echoes is accomplished by reflection, as previously mentioned. When a transmitted wave crosses the boundary of tissues with different wave speeds, refraction causes it to divert from its original direction. When a wave interacts with a structure that is much smaller than its wavelength, such as when it interacts with red blood cells, the result is known as scatter, which is the scattering of the wave in all directions. But absorption is what causes the majority of attenuation. The sound wave's energy is transformed into heat by friction between oscillating tissue particles. However, diagnostic ultrasonography does not generate enough heat to injure the patient's skin.

The ultrasound transducer will only receive a very small amount of energy from the returning echoes, especially from deeper structures, due to the general attenuation through all tissue types and the fact that only a small portion of the wave's energy is reflected at many tissue interfaces, which is then attenuated further as it travels back towards the probe. The ultrasound machine uses a technique called time gain compensation to make up for this energy loss. This produces a more equal image by amplifying those echoes that take longer to return to the transducer.

2.4 Image Resolution

The ability of an imaging system to recognize two distinct locations in space is known as spatial resolution. The ability to discriminate between two structures along the same scan line, that is, in a direction parallel to the beam, is known as axial resolution or depth resolution. This latter type of resolution is only seen when a structure is larger than many of the wavelengths of the ultrasound.

It is important to keep in mind that wavelength and frequency have an inverse relationship, which means that the higher the frequency, the better the axial resolution (shorter the wavelength). To create image of tiny structures, a high-frequency probe is therefore necessary. However, as already mentioned previously, higher frequency waves attenuate more quickly and are more suitable for surface-level structures [1].

The capacity to differentiate two structures that are adjacent and at the same depth is known as lateral resolution. This requires that the beam width be smaller

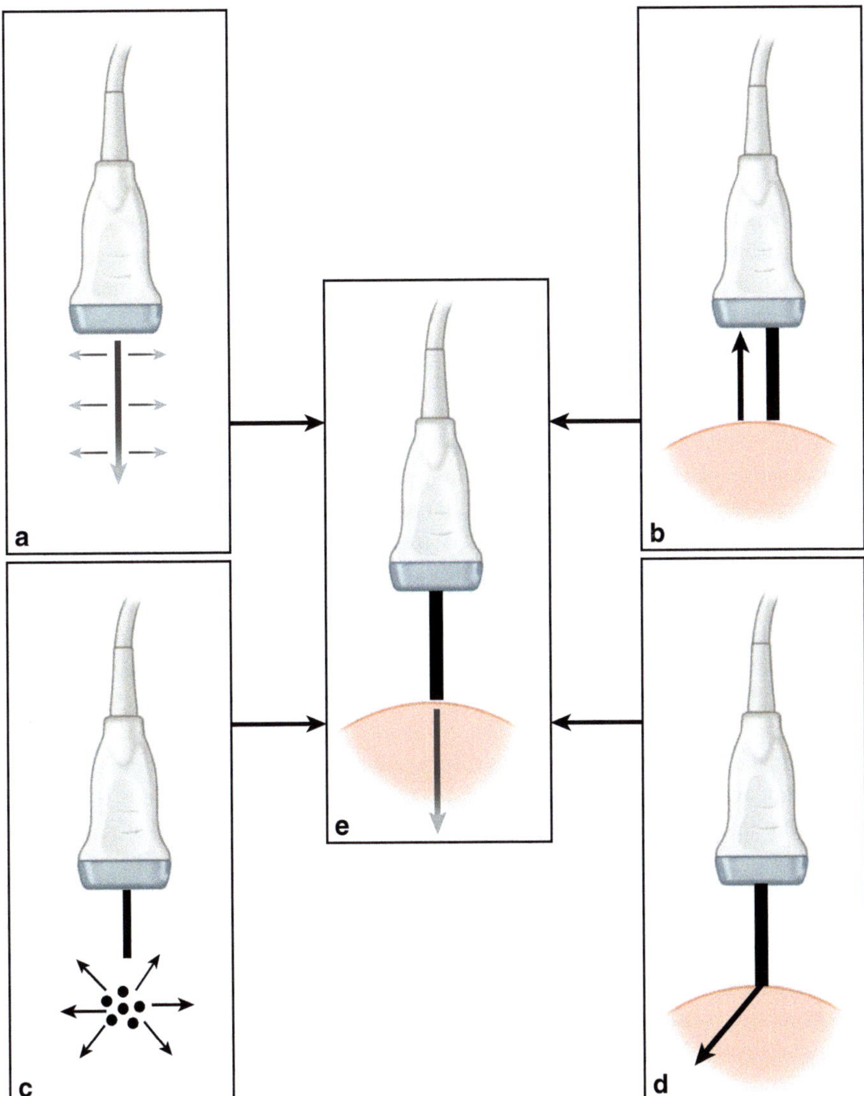

Fig. 2.3 (**a**) Absorption; (**b**) reflection; (**c**) scatter; and (**d**) refractional contribute to the overall attenuation of the ultrasound wave seen in (**e**)

than the separation between the two structures, which is ameliorated with focusing. By taking advantage of the phased array of the probe, a point will be reached where the pulses all arrive together and reinforce each other, allowing the beam to be focused. Practically speaking, it is crucial that the operator places the focal zone accurately during scanning to guarantee the best lateral resolution for evaluating a specific structure.

2.5 Ultrasound Imaging Artifacts

Imaging artifacts are relatively common and may cause misinterpretations, though they may eventually be helpful to in some situations [1, 3].

When sound waves bounce back and forth between two reflective surfaces before reaching back to the transducer, the phenomenon known as **reverberation artifact** (Fig. 2.4a) takes place. Due to the processor's assumption that these echoes are coming from deeper structures, they will follow the original echo in a sequential order and arrive at different times, resulting in a large number of lines that are equally spaced apart.

When sound waves strike a small object, such a tiny air bubble, the result is a phenomenon called **ring-down artifact** (Fig. 2.4b), which causes the object to resonate at the same frequency as ultrasound and create sound. After the initial wave has been reflected back to the transducer, sound is generated. As a result, it will be perceived as a second echo coming from a deeper structure and will appear as a bright line far away from the initial target. Practically speaking, this artifact can be used to help identify air in the biliary tree, for instance. At extremely reflective surfaces, the **mirror artifact** (Fig. 2.4c) appears. A neighboring structure causes the initial beam to reflect from its surface, at which time the original echo is returned to the highly reflecting surface before being reflected back to the transducer. This is taken to mean that something is coming back from a deeper structure that is thought to be on the other side of the reflective surface. Traditionally, this occurs at the diaphragm.

When the ultrasonic beam strikes a very attenuating or highly reflecting surface, **posterior acoustic shadowing** (Fig. 2.4d) takes place. Because there is little to no through transmission, there is darkness beneath the surface. This makes it harder to visualize any structure up to this point. Practically speaking, this artifact can aid in locating calcified structures such as gallstones and renal calculi.

When the ultrasound beam travels through a weakly attenuating structure, such as the fluid in a straightforward cyst or the urine in the bladder, **posterior acoustic enhancement** (Fig. 2.4e) takes place. As more of the original beam's energy reaches the structures behind the cyst, they will seem brighter, and an echo with more energy will be reflected back to the probe as a result.

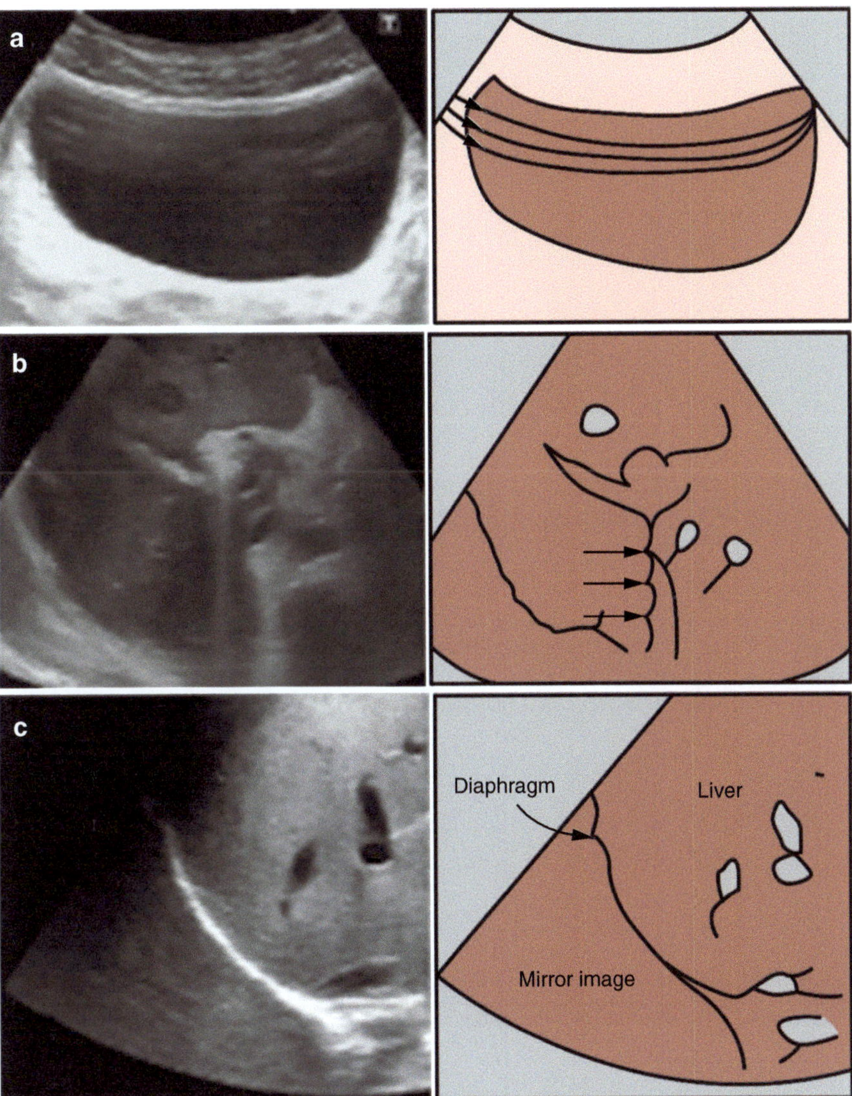

Fig. 2.4 Ultrasound artifacts. (**a**) Reverberation artifact evenly spaced lines in the bladder. (**b**) Ring-down artifact e bright white line caused by air within the biliary tree. (**c**) Mirror artifact e liver "reflected" on the other side of the diaphragm. (**d**) Posterior acoustic shadowing e caused by two gallstones in the gallbladder. (**e**) Posterior acoustic enhancement e due to simple liver cyst

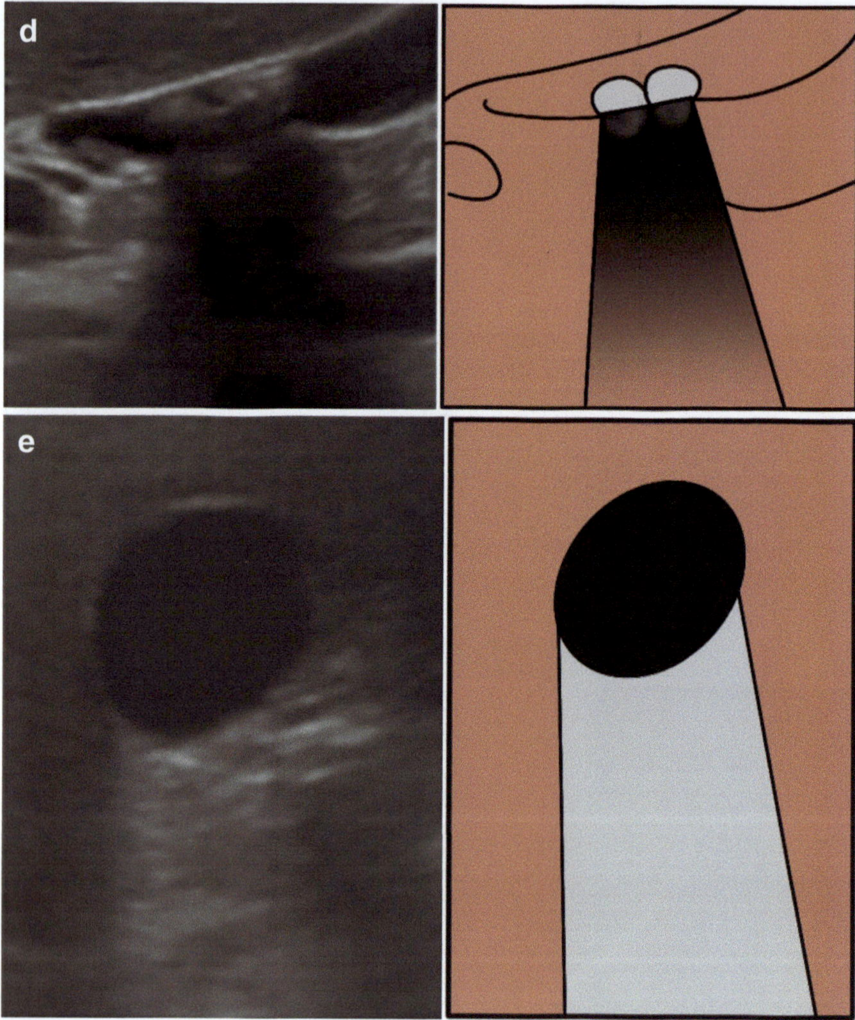

Fig. 2.4 (continued)

2.6   Doppler Effect

The Doppler effect describes the change in frequency of an incident wave that occurs when it is reflected at a moving interface, which is why the pitch of a moving vehicle's horn appears to change as it approaches and passes a stationary observer [4]. Figure 2.5 features a common example that illustrates the Doppler effect. Everyone is aware that when we pause to listen to an ambulance siren as it passes, the pitch of the siren changes. The frequency that reaches you increases as the ambulance draws near and decreases as it passes by, and this is a classic demonstration of the Doppler effect.

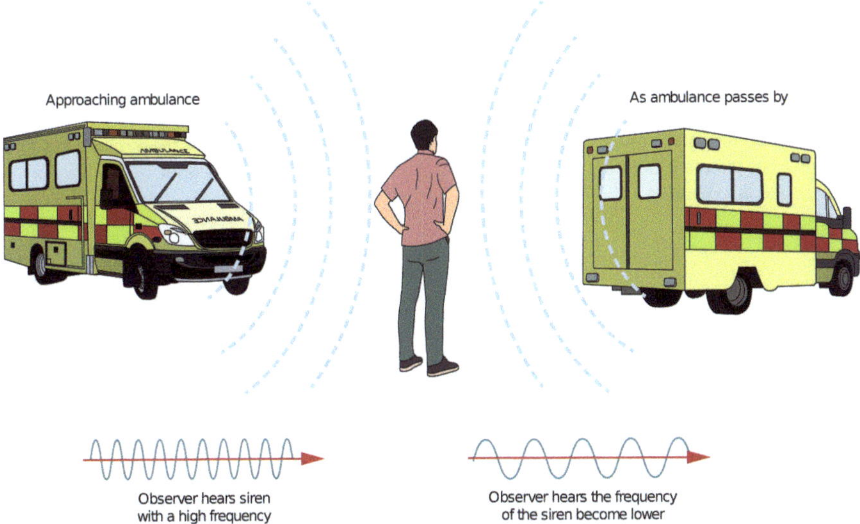

Fig. 2.5 The Doppler effect affects the relative frequency of an ambulance's siren as it passes by. In contrast to the passing ambulance's siren, which has a lower frequency, the incoming ambulance's siren displays a higher sound frequency

The mathematician and physicist Christian Johann Doppler, who first identified this phenomenon in 1842 by examining light from stars, is honored by having his name attached to the Doppler principle. He showed that the motion of the stars in relation to the earth is what gives them their colorful look. Either a red shift or a blue change in the light's frequency resulted from this relative motion. The Doppler effect, which affects both light and sound waves, describes this change in the measured frequency of waves from moving sources [1, 4].

When a sound-producing object is traveling in the same direction as the waves, the sound waves are compressed. As a result, shorter wavelengths are received by the listener (observer). The listener, however, detects a change in frequency after the source of sound has past them and the waves are now traveling in the opposite direction (away from them). As a result, the wavelength lengthens, and the waves move in the opposite direction. By examining the relative frequency shifts of the received echoes caused by the movement of red blood cells, this Doppler effect is used in ultrasound applications to detect blood flow [4, 5].

2.7   The Doppler Effect Applied to Diagnostic Ultrasound

For instance, blood flow can be studied using the Doppler effect in diagnostic imaging, which gives the operator three details to ascertain: (1) the presence or absence of blood flow as well as blood flow's (2) direction and (3) velocity.

Doppler ultrasound is transmitted and received by the transducer. The transducer picks up the returning backscattered echoes from blood when using Doppler to

Fig. 2.6 Examination of a blood vessel with an ultrasonic transducer. Sending a Doppler signal at frequency Ft while detecting the backscattered signals from the red blood cells inside the vessel at frequency Fr

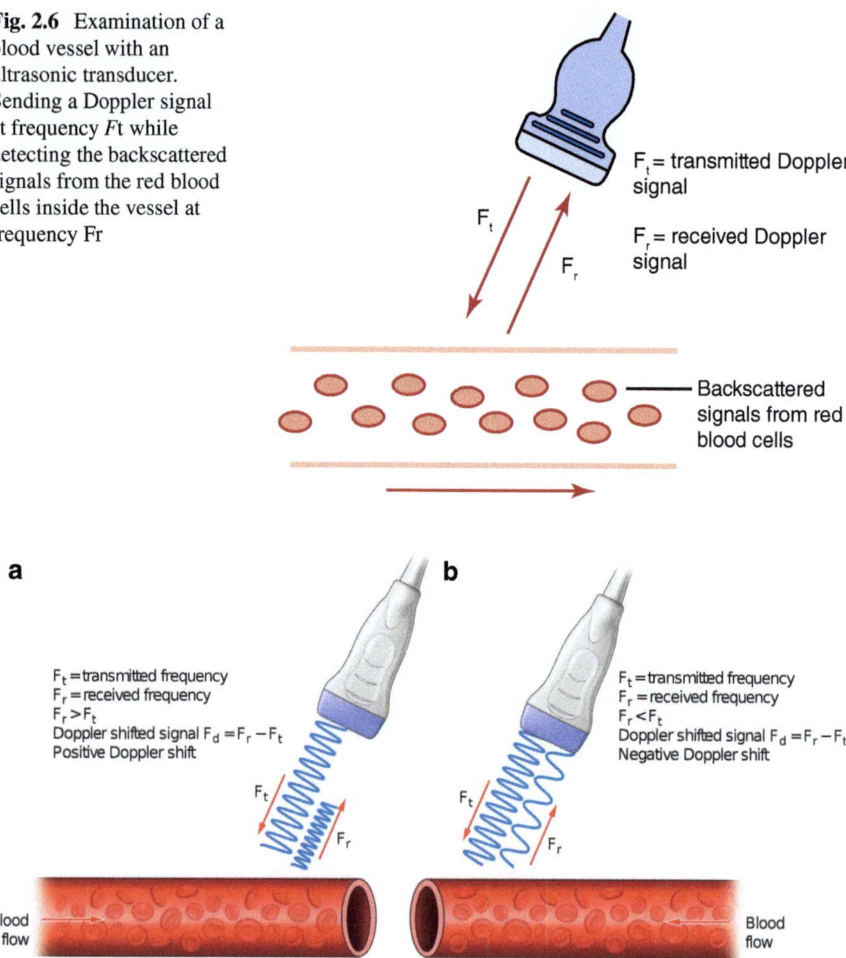

Fig. 2.7 Doppler signal shifts in blood flow traveling in two directions: (**a**) towards the transducer and (**b**) away from the transducer

examine blood flow in the body. The computer then processes these backscattered signals (Fr) to identify any frequency changes by contrasting these signals with the transmitted Doppler signals (Ft). The amount and direction of blood flow will determine two factors that will affect the frequency shift that is detected, as shown in Fig. 2.6.

Consider the configuration shown in Fig. 2.7 in which the Ft-frequency Doppler signal is sent by the transducer. The transducer picks up the backscattered signals from the red blood cells inside the vessel at a frequency Fr after the transmitted Doppler signal reaches a blood vessel. By taking the sent signal Ft and the received signal Fr and subtracting them, the Doppler frequency shift (Fd) may be determined.

Doppler shifted signals are positive when blood flow is flowing towards the transducer and negative when blood flow is moving away from the transducer. Blood moving toward and away from the transducer causes a change in the received backscattered signals, which is shown in Fig. 2.7 along with the accompanying Doppler shifts.

The relative direction of the blood flow with regard to the Doppler beam in Fig. 2.7a is in the direction of the transducer. Blood flow traveling towards the transducer in this configuration results in received signals (Fr) that have a higher frequency than the broadcast beam (Ft). By deducting Ft from Fr, one may determine the Doppler shifted signal (Fd), which results in a positive Doppler shifted signal. Figure 2.7b, on the other hand, shows blood flow that is flowing away from the transducer and the Doppler beam. This configuration generates received signals (Fr) that are lower in frequency than the sent beam due to blood flow flowing away from the transducer (Ft). This time, a negative Doppler shifted signal is produced by the Doppler shifted frequencies (Fr Ft). The transmission frequency (Ft) is equal to the received frequency when there is no flow or movement observed (Fr). There are no Doppler shifted signals as a result of Fr = Ft and Fd = Fr Ft = 0.

The amplitude of the backscattered echoes from blood must be understood to be substantially weaker than those from soft tissue and organ interfaces, which are employed to construct our B-mode anatomical pictures. Blood can cause the backscattered signal's amplitude to be reduced by a factor of 100–1000. In order to ensure that these signals can be identified and processed, highly sensitive and complex hardware and processing software are needed.

The detected Doppler shifted signal (Fd) and the blood flow velocity (V) are mathematically related, as shown by the Doppler equation:

$$F_d = \frac{2 F_t V \cos\theta}{c},\tag{2.1}$$

where: Fd = Doppler shifted signal, Ft = transmitted Doppler frequency, c = the propagation speed of ultrasound in soft tissue (1540 ms^{-1}), V = velocity of the moving blood, θ = the angle between the Doppler ultrasound beam and the direction of blood flow, 2 = the number 2 is a constant indicating that the Doppler beam must travel to the moving target and then back to the transducer.

2.7.1   Relationship Between Doppler Shifted Signal (Fd) and Blood Flow Velocity (V)

The Doppler equation (Eq. 2.1) shows that the blood flow velocity (V) and the Doppler shifted signal (Fd) are related. Blood flow velocity (V) and the Doppler shifted signal (Fd) are directly proportional, meaning that higher flow velocities result in bigger Doppler shifted signals and lower flow velocities result in smaller

Doppler shifted signals. The Doppler equation can be adjusted (see Eq. 2.2) to determine blood flow velocities (V), which can then be processed and displayed if we can identify and quantify the value of Fd.

$$V = \frac{F_{\mathrm{d}}c}{2F_{\mathrm{t}}\cos\theta}.$$

(2.2)

2.7.2 Significance of the Doppler Angle (θ)

An operator must be aware of the significance of the angle of insonation (θ) between the Doppler beam and the direction of blood flow in vessels since ultrasound devices can determine Doppler shifted frequencies over a wide range of angles. The Doppler shifted signal's evolution as the Doppler beam angle varies is depicted visually in Fig. 2.8.

A positive Doppler shifted signal can be detected when the Doppler beam is pointing towards the direction of blood flow, but a negative Doppler shifted signal can be seen when the Doppler beam is pointing in the opposite direction. The size of the Doppler shifted signal increases with the angle between the blood vessel and Doppler beam. As the Doppler beam angle approaches a 90° angle, very tiny signals are generated.

Table 2.1 shows the relationship between the angle of the Doppler beam (θ) and the value of $\cos\theta$. The value of $\cos\theta$ varies with the angle from 0 to 1. When $\theta = 0°$, $\cos\theta = 1$, and when $\theta = 90°$, $\cos\theta = 0$.

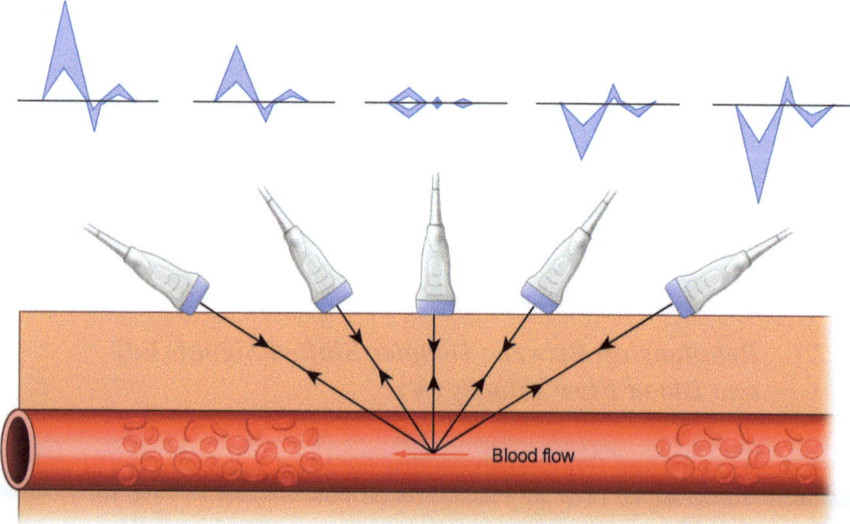

Fig. 2.8 Graphical demonstration of how the angle of the insonating Doppler beam and the Doppler shifted frequency relate to one another

Table 2.1 $\cos\theta$ variations at different insonation angles

Angle θ	Value of $\cos\theta$
0	1
30	0.87
45	0.71
60	0.5
75	0.26
90	0

A Doppler beam angle of 0° is represented by the highest value of $\cos\theta$

The largest value of $\cos\theta$, and consequently the highest value of the Doppler shifted signal (Fd), occurs at an angle of 0° with a constant flow velocity (V). This is equivalent to a Doppler beam parallel to the vessel, which is extremely difficult to achieve in clinical practice. In theory, when $\theta = 90°$, the blood flow is perpendicular to the Doppler beam, $\cos 90° = 0$, and no Doppler shifted signals are registered.

To obtain accurate Doppler shifted signals, it is crucial in practice to use a Doppler beam angle between 30° and 60° while measuring blood flow. Ideally examiners were supposed to be kept around 60° and should keep in mind that 90° does not produce any Doppler shifted signals. Larger Doppler shifted frequencies are produced by faster flows and narrower angles, but not by stronger Doppler shift signals.

2.8 Doppler Modes

The first mode made available in Doppler ultrasound technology was the spectral Doppler. On the y-axis of this Doppler mode's graph is the spectrum of flow velocities, while time is observed on the x-axis. As a result, it is possible to measure a variety of blood flow characteristics using spectral mode, in which peak systolic velocity, end diastolic velocity, and resistive index are applicable to hemodynamic evaluation. Later on Doppler color flow imaging was created, also known as color Doppler (CD) mode. Real-time ultrasound imaging and the Doppler effect are actually combined in the CD technology.

In CD mode, the Doppler technique's data is incorporated as a color signal into the B-mode, which provides images in gray scale. On top of B-mode imaging, real-time flow data in the form of a color signal is superimposed. The flow direction is indicated by colors. Blue often denotes flow away from the transducer and red typically denotes flow towards the transducer.

The most recent Doppler mode, Power Doppler (PD) mode, has been used in US technology since the 1990s. When compared to CD, which shows the mean Doppler shift, PD shows the power of the Doppler shift in each cell, which solely shows signal intensity (i.e., amount of red blood cells flowing). Additionally, PD is more susceptible to motion artifacts than CD, is essentially angle independent, and shows weaker definition of the flow profile and pulsatility. Many high-end US machines now have CD modes that are far more sensitive to detecting flow at the microvascular level [1, 5, 6].

2.9   Doppler Parameters

Optimal adjustment of CD or PD Doppler setting is essential to enhance the quality of Doppler US assessment. To achieve the best sensitivity for detecting flow with or without minimal artifacts, Doppler settings should be modified according to each specific scenario. These parameters vary depending on the depth of the examined anatomic area and are dependent on US equipment. For each anatomical areas such as deep, intermediate, or superficial tissues, pre-established presets with the proper Doppler parameters may be prerecorded for prompt use when required, which is highly useful and saves time in everyday practice. The most relevant Doppler settings that examiners should be aware of are described below.

2.9.1   Focusing

The focal point should be positioned at the same level as the target region, just like in B-mode.

2.9.2   Doppler Frequency

Doppler frequencies should generally be employed at high levels for superficial anatomical regions and at low levels for deep anatomical regions. However, most US machines will determine the best frequencies that should be ideally used at various depths.

2.9.3   Pulse Repetition Frequency (PRF)

In both color and spectral Doppler imaging, PRF also known as velocity scale plays a crucial role in determining the frequency range exhibited. If the dynamic range is too wide, low velocity signals may be missed. This phenomenon might mimic an area of thrombosis, especially in low flow veins like the portal vein, if the scale is set too high. Doppler is more sensitive to detecting low velocity flow from tiny arteries in inflammatory illnesses when the PRF is low. However, an excessively low PRF may cause motion artifacts at the slightest movement of patient, probe, artery wall, or patient voice. The interpretation of genuine flow in US photos can be quite challenging due to these artifacts. Therefore, optimal PRF values are those as low as possible, which allow detection low velocity flows without significant motion artifacts.

Moreover, the dynamic range may be insufficient to accurately display high-velocity data if the velocity scale is set too low, which may eventually lead to aliasing, an artifact that will be explained in this chapter.

2.9.4   Doppler Gain

The Doppler sensitivity is improved with increasing Doppler gain, up to a certain point in which noise artifacts start to be detected. Therefore, examiners should operate with the highest Doppler gain possible without random noise being detected. In other words, color gain should be set just below the level at which color noise is developed. It is important to mention that the utilized US device has a significant influence on the optimal Doppler gain.

2.9.5   Doppler Angle

Doppler US produces the greatest signals with best spectra when the motion is parallel to the beam as opposed to grayscale US imaging, in which the best image is produced perpendicularly to the US beam. A Doppler angle of 90° does not show evidence of flow, since there is no component of the frequency shift that is directed back toward the transducer. Therefore, angle adjustments are necessary for any Doppler angle other than zero to account for the signal component that is not parallel to the beam. The Doppler beam angle must always be kept as low as possible since the larger the Doppler angle, the more correction is required and the more chance of error. Because the angle correction errors rise by up to 20–30% with increasing Doppler angles, the ideal value should always be less than 60°.

2.9.6   Wall Filter

Doppler's sensitivity for detecting flow in small vessels or conduits is increased if low wall filters are applied.

2.9.7 Doppler Box

The region of interest, which should contain the examined anatomical structure and an adequate view of adjacent tissues, should be highlighted with the appropriate color box size. Sometimes if Doppler boxes are not adequately placed, reverberation artifacts may be caused.

2.9.8 Sample Volume

The Doppler frequency shifts are measured from a specific sample volume in a three-dimensional space. The sample volume is characterized according to the Doppler mode. In power or color Doppler mode, sample volume is represented by color box, while in pulsed wave Doppler, it is characterized by the cursor that is placed inside the vessel. Although the sample appears to be a flat box on the image, it actually also operates in a third dimension that extends into and out of the image's plane and may reach 1 cm or more in thickness, depending on frequency and depth.

Because of friction and turbulence, blood flow in large vessels is not uniform, being typically faster in the center and slower near the wall. Due to the inclusion of the usual turbulence and slower velocities around the vessel margins in a excessively large sample that covers the whole vessel lumen, spectral Doppler may result in spectral broadening, which may be incorrectly interpreted as post stenotic turbulence. On the other hand, the measured velocity will be too low if the spectral sample is too tiny and not located where the strongest flow is. A discontinuous Doppler signal with loss of the diastolic signal in each cycle may come from a small sample volume or a mobile vessel. The ideal sample volume size for routine assessment of a vessel is approximately two thirds of the vessel width placed in its center.

2.9.9 Color Priority

When detecting blood flow is the main goal of the ultrasound examination, this setting should be prioritized over grayscale priority.

2.10 Most Common Doppler Artifacts

Doppler artifacts can be categorized into three main groups: (1) those caused by technical issues, such as aliasing, improper Doppler angles with no flow, blooming, and partial volume artifact; (2) those secondary to patient anatomy, such as mirror image artifact, flash artifact, and "pseudoflow"; and (3) those resulting from machine factors, such as edge artifact and twinkle artifact [3].

2.10.1   Aliasing

Aliasing is an artifact caused by ambiguity in measuring high Doppler frequency shifts. When using a pulsed wave Doppler system, it is necessary to wait for the echo from the area of interest before transmitting the next pulse to ensure that samples come from only a specific depth. This restricts the rate at which pulses can be generated, with a lower PRF required for greater depth. The PRF also determines the deepest point from which unambiguous data can be obtained.

Aliasing occurs when the PRF is less than twice the maximum frequency shift produced by moving the target (Nyquist limit). In other words, when PRF is less than twice of the actual frequency shift, lower frequency shifts may start to appear, thus generating aliasing effects.

Signals from deep abdominal arteries are prone to aliasing if high velocities are present due to the need for lower PRFs to reach deep vessels. In practice, aliasing is usually obvious. Aliasing can be reduced by increasing the PRF, decreasing the frequency shift by increasing the Doppler angle, or using a lower-frequency Doppler transducer (Fig. 2.9).

2.10.2   Blooming Artifact

The color extends from inside the vessel and "bleeds" past the wall into surrounding surfaces, giving rise to the term "color bleed." Since the color US image is actually two images—the color and the gray scale—superimposed, color bleed may happen. Depending on how the parameters are adjusted, the color section of the image may thus go beyond the actual grayscale vessel margin. The most prevalent cause of this extension, which typically happens deep inside the arteries, is unusually high gain settings. The information inside the vessel (i.e., the partial thrombus) may be

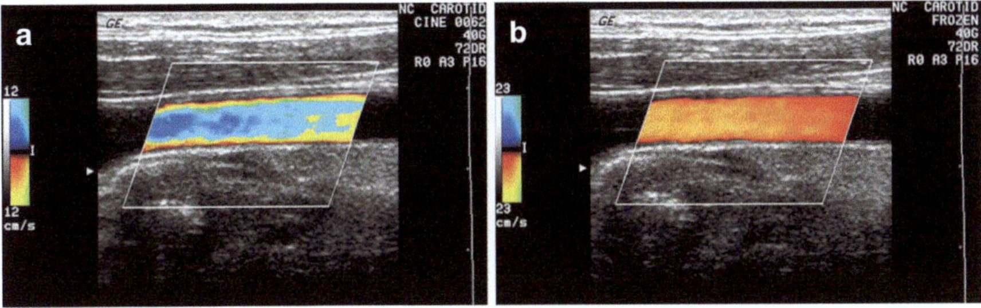

Fig. 2.9 Color Doppler aliasing. (**a**) Longitudinal CDUS image of CCA directed away from transducer should be red with maximum central velocity displayed as bright yellow. Instead, color scale "wraps around" and colors are displayed sequentially from red and yellow adjacent to wall to light blue and then dark blue in central lumen. PRF range is 12 cm s^{-1}. (**b**) At proper scale range of 23 cm s^{-1}, color display no longer aliases and flow direction is depicted appropriately

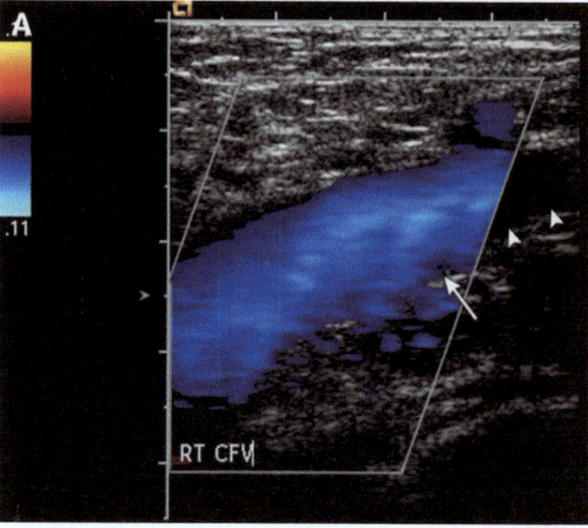

Fig. 2.10 Blooming artifact. (A) Longitudinal CDUS image of right common femoral vein (CFV) shows blooming artifact deep to vessel, displaying color (arrow) beyond vessel wall (arrowheads). Scale is low at 0.11 and gain high at 50

"written over" and concealed, which an undesirable effect should be avoided as much as possible (Fig. 2.10).

2.10.3   Directional Ambiguity

A spectral Doppler tracing with the waveform exhibited with roughly equal amplitude above and below the baseline in a mirror image pattern is referred to as having directional ambiguity or ambiguous flow direction. Small vessels, especially those that might be moving in and out of the imaging plane, are more likely to exhibit this pattern, which is created when the beam intercepts the vessel at a 90° angle (Fig. 2.11). True bidirectional flow should not be confused with directional ambiguity. Blood really flows in two directions; in the latter scenario, it is found, for example, in the neck of a pseudoaneurysm. The fact that the flow changes direction within a single cardiac cycle from one direction to the other is a key indicator. Diastolic flow reversal is a different type of bidirectional flow that happens in conditions of high resistance organ flow (such as twisting, venous thrombosis, or other sources of parenchymal edema). True bidirectional flow is never concurrently symmetric above and below the baseline, which distinguishes it from an indeterminate direction spectral tracing. Throughout the cardiac cycle, the flow direction changes.

2.10.4   Artifact of Partial Volume

A non-infinitely thin slice thickness causes partial volume artifacts. Echoes and Doppler signals may be obtained from items that are partially inside and partially outside of the slice, analogous to cutting a strawberry in a piece of fruit cake

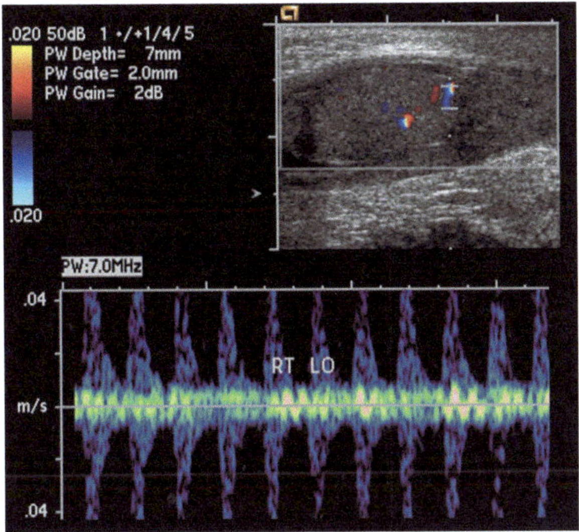

Fig. 2.11 Longitudinal CDUS image through infant testis shows arterial spectral Doppler waveform with equal amplitude above and below baseline, yielding an indeterminate flow direction. This occurs most often in small vessels

partially through. The slice resembles a strawberry when seen from one side. No strawberry appears to be visible when viewed from the opposite angle. Echoes can arise inside anechoic structures, and Doppler signals can be obtained in a location where no vessels are visible in gray scale because the signals in the US slice are added together, attributing the created echoes to structures in the supposed "thin" scan plane. For instance, echoes from gas in the duodenum may appear inside the gallbladder on a longitudinal grayscale image and resemble stones or polyps; however, if you rotate the transducer and image from the transverse plane, the gas is obviously adjacent to the gallbladder and not inside it. These transducer-related aberrations, which mostly affect high-frequency, tightly curved, convex, linear arrays employed in endocavitary probes, rely on the size of the crystal elements and the spacing between the elements of the array.

2.10.5   *Pseudoflow*

The definition of pseudoflow is the existence of fluid flow that is not blood. Pseudoflow can simulate actual blood flow using color or power Doppler US, but there is not a real vessel that actually contains the fluid. As long as the fluid motion persists, the color or power Doppler signal appears. Without Doppler spectrum analysis, these artifacts can be mistaken for flow. An average arterial or venous waveform is not visible on the spectral Doppler tracing. Bladder jets, amniotic fluid, and ascites are all examples of spontaneous pseudoflow.

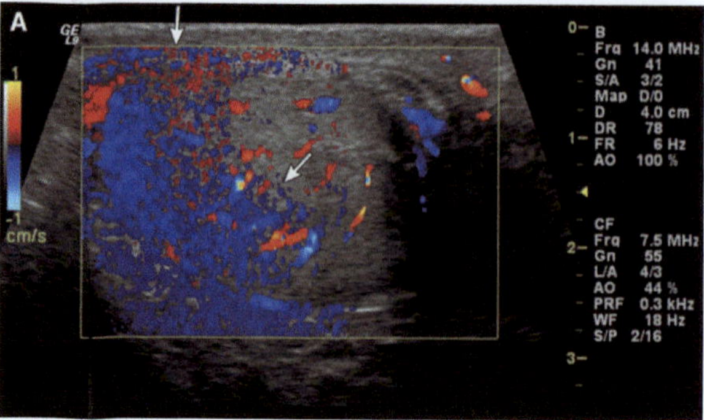

Fig. 2.12 Flash artifact: patient motion. Longitudinal CDUS through the left lobe of liver with flash artifact (arrows) produced by respiratory motion

2.10.6 Flashing

Flash artifacts are random bursts of color that obscure grayscale images. Object or transducer motion can generate this phenomenon (Fig. 2.12). Flash artifacts are more common in the left lobe of the liver (due to heart pulse) and in hypoechoic regions, such as cysts or fluid collections. Cremasteric reflex may also generate this artifact on testicles. Flash artifacts indicate fluidity in solid-appearing material. Power Doppler is more prone to flash artifacts than color flow Doppler because more frames are averaged to form the image.

2.10.7 Mirror Artifact

The mirror image artifact displays items on opposite sides of a strong reflector. The reflector (diaphragm, pleural surface, or aortic wall) transmits some echoes to a second reflector before returning them to the transducer. The machine "straightens out" multipath echoes by assuming they come from the initial transducer beam and a distance proportional to the actual duration of flight, resulting in deeper echoes than they should be. The outcome is a virtual object similar to the original image, hence the word "mirror." Gray scale, color, power, and spectral Doppler may form mirror images.

2.10.8 Edging

In imaging, edge artifact is the Doppler signal produced at the edge of a strong, smooth, specular reflector. It appears as persistent color along the rim of calcified structures, such as gallstones or cortical bone, and unless spectral tracing is obtained, it may be mistaken for vascularity. Any echogenic surface, including artificial structures such catheters and Foley balloons, may produce edge artifact. The Doppler spectrum, which is a straight-line pattern with equal lengths above and below the baseline and represents noise rather than flow, is the diagnostic feature. Due to the

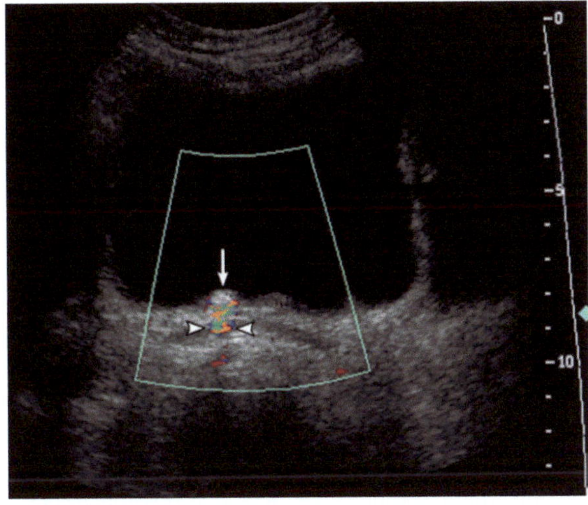

Fig. 2.13 Twinkling artifact. Longitudinal image of bladder shows typical ureterovesical junction stone (arrow) with posterior shadow

system's heightened sensitivity, these artifacts are more common at low PRF or velocity scale, though they can also be caused by a low wall filter setting.

2.10.9 Twinkling

It is defined as color Doppler signals that resemble motion or flow behind a stationary brightly reflecting interface. The sparkling artifact is induced by renal calculi, bladder calcification, and gallbladder cholesterol crystals. The twinkling Doppler is a mosaic of changing colors near an echogenic reflector (Fig. 2.13). The twinkling signal can be detected based on color-write priority and grayscale gain. As color-write priority falls, more gray scale is presented and sparkling artifact reduces. Gray scale has less impact at high color-write priorities. These parameters vary by ultrasound machine and by brand. Twinkling artifacts can help identify stones like grayscale shadowing. Small stones without a substantial echo or acoustic shadow can cause a sparkling artifact. The key to the twinkling artifact is that the color behind the calcification and the concurrent Doppler spectral tracing indicate noise, not flow.

2.11 Tips and Tricks for Better Clinical Practice Using Doppler Methodology

The artifacts mentioned in the "Doppler Artifacts" section are mostly associated with the production of Doppler signals by nonvascular structures or fluids. Knowing that they can happen, understanding the typical sources of their genesis and locations, and recognizing the nonvascular Doppler spectrum they produce, which may eventually establish the diagnosis, are all essential to recognizing them.

The more frequent issues in daily clinical practice are excessive flow, as they may eventually mimic thrombi or insufficient flow and lead to a mistaken diagnosis of thrombosis.

In most cases, color bleed or aliasing in a vessel that ordinarily does not have it serves as an indicator of excessive flow. By increasing the scale (PRF) or lowering the gain, this issue can be fixed. Another frequent imaging issue arises when continuous flow is observed from a conduit segment and flow is presumed to be the same across the remainder of the lumen. A partial thrombus or atheromatous plaque may not be imaged if it is not centered in the imaging plane, a problem that typically arises in longitudinal vascular imaging. Ideally, the examiner should always image in two planes as a fail-safe in case the incorrect settings are not noticed. With this precaution even if the color-write priority is set too high or the imaging plane is not centered and the thrombus is overwritten in the long axis of the vessel, the clot can still be seen in the short axis plane.

The other frequent issue is insufficient flow, which resembles thrombosis. The Doppler angle should be as modest as possible to begin with. It is rarely easy to get signals of flow at 90° to the probe. The scale needs to be calibrated for the vessel you are investigating. A scale that is too high eliminates the vessels' slow flow.

Low frequency for deep structures and high frequency for superficial ones are the proper frequencies to use. If the Doppler frequency does not automatically default to the right frequency, it may be necessary to reduce it manually because the frequency required to illustrate color flow Doppler is typically lower than the frequency required for grayscale imaging. If they are set too high, frequency filters and other techniques meant to reduce color tissue noise may stop displaying slow-moving blood. In general, shrinking the color box increases the frame rate and decreases the sample size, improving the sensitivity and resolution of the color image as a whole. The color-write priority can also be manually or automatically determined. If the color-write priority is set too low, flow could be overlooked. Conversely, if the color-write priority is set too high, the sensitivity for color flow can be prioritized so that color appears when no vessel was seen on grayscale imaging.

Table 2.2 provides a summary of useful recommendations for enhancing a color Doppler test.

Table 2.2 Guidelines for an optimal color flow Doppler examination

Box 1: Guidelines for an optimal color flow Doppler examination
• Adjust the gain and filter settings to obtain an optimal color signal and minimal color noise
• Adjust the velocity scale (PRF) and baseline according to the flow conditions. A low scale is used for low flows and velocities; however, it may produce aliasing. A high scale reduces aliasing but is less sensitive for slow flows
• Obtain an optimal Doppler angle by adjusting the beam steering and probe position. The angle should be 60° or less if velocity measurements are to be made
• The color flow box should be kept as small as possible to allow better frame rate for better resolution and sensitivity
• Adjust the pulsed Doppler sample volume size appropriately (two thirds of the vessel diameter) to obtain accurate velocities
• Avoid transducer motion

2.12 Conclusions

In conclusion, the chapter on the principles of Doppler ultrasound has provided a comprehensive understanding of this powerful diagnostic imaging technique. Doppler ultrasound has revolutionized the field of medical imaging by allowing healthcare professionals to assess blood flow patterns and velocity in real-time. By utilizing the Doppler effect, which is based on the frequency shift of sound waves reflected from moving objects, Doppler ultrasound enables the noninvasive evaluation of various vascular conditions. To optimize imaging and make appropriate clinical determinations, it is instrumental that users understand the principles of different Doppler modalities and how Doppler information is processed.

References

1. Rumack CM, Levine D. Diagnostic ultrasound. Elsevier Health Sciences; 2017.
2. Hangiandreou NJ. AAPM/RSNA physics tutorial for residents: topics in US: B-mode US: basic concepts and new technology. Radiographics. 2003;23(4):1019–33.
3. Feldman MK, Katyal S, Blackwood MS. US artifacts. Radiographics. 2009;29(4):1179–89.
4. Taylor K, Holland S. Doppler US. Part I. Basic principles, instrumentation, and pitfalls. Radiology. 1990;174(2):297–307.
5. Rubens DJ, Bhatt S, Nedelka S, Cullinan J. Doppler artifacts and pitfalls. Radiol Clin. 2006;44(6):805–35.
6. Campbell SC, Cullinan JA, Rubens DJ. Slow flow or no flow? Color and power Doppler US pitfalls in the abdomen and pelvis. Radiographics. 2004;24(2):497–506.

Chapter 3
Minimum Requirements for an Ultrasound Machine, Basic Setup, and Adjustments for Penile Hemodynamic Studies

3.1 Introduction

Ultrasonography is a widespread and crucial diagnostic instrument in the medical field. Due to sophisticated equipment and automatic picture optimization, ultrasonic imaging takes little technical and physical understanding to be implemented in current practice. For optimal image adjustment and documentation, however, a thorough understanding of the device's function repertoire and underlying mechanisms is required. The goal should always be to achieve the best possible image quality for medical, research, and even aesthetic purposes [1].

Doppler ultrasound is an essential imaging tool that is usually used in conjunction with conventional B-mode sonography. It enables noninvasive and non-ionizing assessment of vascular blood flow. Compared to the axial imaging techniques such as magnetic resonance imaging (MRI) or computed tomography (CT), ultrasound (US) Doppler imaging depends heavily on the examiner's skills and expertise. A thorough understanding of anatomy, as well as ideal instrument and image settings, is required for achieving accurate and trustworthy US diagnoses.

Optimal US device settings in a structured and practical manner for an ideal penile hemodynamic evaluation will be discussed in this chapter, with a focus on Pulsed Wave Doppler (PW) US and color Doppler ultrasound (CD). While CD shows the architecture of blood vessels in a particular field of view within the US image as well as the direction of flow, PW offers information on blood flow characteristics at a specific spot of the cavernous artery (i.e., velocity of blood cells) [2].

© The Author(s), under exclusive license to Springer Nature Switzerland AG 2024
E. d. P. Miranda, F. Carneiro, *Penile Color Duplex-Doppler Ultrasound in Erectile Dysfunction Diagnosis and Management*,
https://doi.org/10.1007/978-3-031-55649-4_3

3.2 Ultrasound Machine and Transducer

Before discussing the PW Doppler and color Doppler set up for the penile examination, we must first establish the minimal requirements for an ultrasound apparatus. It is also important to consider the selection of an adequate transducer that will be utilized for the penile Doppler hemodynamic examination. It is the authors understanding that pocket ultrasound equipment are insufficient to conduct a high-quality, in-depth investigation. These machines are suitable for point-of-care ultrasonography (POCUS), which entails targeted and rapid application for prompt diagnosis and action (interventional procedures) and therefore should not be applied for producing reliable evaluations of penile hemodynamics. These devices have only a few configuration options, a more complicated and less intuitive user interface, and typically poor frame rates, which makes Doppler modes slow. With these limited resources, it is almost impossible to achieve accurate studies in a consistent basis. Regarding transducers, the authors suggest those with a minimum frequency of 12 MHz.

In summary, examiners may be able to conduct a quality examination with the aid of new portable ultrasound devices from a variety of manufacturers or conventional and fixed ultrasound machines that provide these minimum quality requirements. On the other hand, it is also important to bear in mind that in the majority of obsolete machines, the Doppler software is outdated and makes penile hemodynamic studies even more challenging, making newer devices preferable.

3.3 Spectral or Pulse Wave (PW) Doppler Ultrasound

Fast Fourier Transformation is used by spectral Doppler modalities (PW) to average the differences between sent and received frequencies over a set amount of time and show these frequency changes as a velocity range.

PW systems use the same crystal to transmit and receive a series of pulses. In PW, the examiner defines a small "sample volume" or "Doppler gate" in the B-mode picture. Only Doppler shifts inside the sample volume area are recorded. PW is a method for measuring flow velocities in cavernous vessels in which the precise location of evaluation can be determined. On the ultrasound scanner console, PW can be activated by pressing the respective button on the interface [3, 4].

3.3.1 PWD Parameter Adjustment

To get the best image adjustment in PW for evaluation of penile Doppler, the following crucial factors must be taken into account:

3.3.1.1 Transmission Frequency

The B-mode or color Doppler frequency has no bearing on the spectral Doppler frequency. The examiner maintains spectral Doppler flow sensitivity in cavernous vessels by adjusting it. The transducer preset must be set to small parts/superficial structures evaluation (i.e., testicle evaluation preset). Higher transmission frequencies should be used for penile vessels as those are superficial structures (12–18 MHz).

3.3.1.2 Pulse Repetition Frequency (PRF)/Scale

Pulse repetition frequency (PRF) refers to the number of sound pulses emitted per second by the transducer. The transmission frequency has no bearing on the PRF. The PRF, which establishes the range or scale (in cm/s) in which flow can be represented without aliasing on ultrasound instruments, is frequently referred to as the (velocity) scale. According to the so-called Nyquist limit, if the Doppler frequency shift of a flow is less than half the pulse repetition frequency (PRF), then the flow velocity being presented will be accurate.

The term "aliasing" refers to the occurrence in which the high-velocity portions of a spectral curve are truncated and displayed below the baseline in the countercurrent direction (Fig. 3.1). It occurs when the maximum flow velocity in a given Doppler gate experiences a frequency shift more than 50% of the PRF. Therefore, if the maximum flow velocities do not exceed the velocity range displayed on the screen, the optimal PRF setting has been achieved. However, the depth localization of the sample volume restricts the maximum PRF. Some flow velocities are so extreme that using a machine set to its default settings makes it impossible to measure them.

Options for enhancing the test in these circumstances include the following:

- Optimizing the probe position making it close to the cavernous vessels.
- Choosing a more appropriated transmission frequency.
- Extending the scope.
- Adjusting the baseline.
- Establishing a greater angle between the vessel and the Doppler beam.

As the velocities of the cavernous arteries vary over a wide range, we propose that the scale be set to a range of approximately 50 cm/s above the baseline, with fine adjustments made as necessary.

3.3.1.3 Baseline

The baseline must be established with the intention of showing an appropriate velocity scale and maximizing the use of the image.

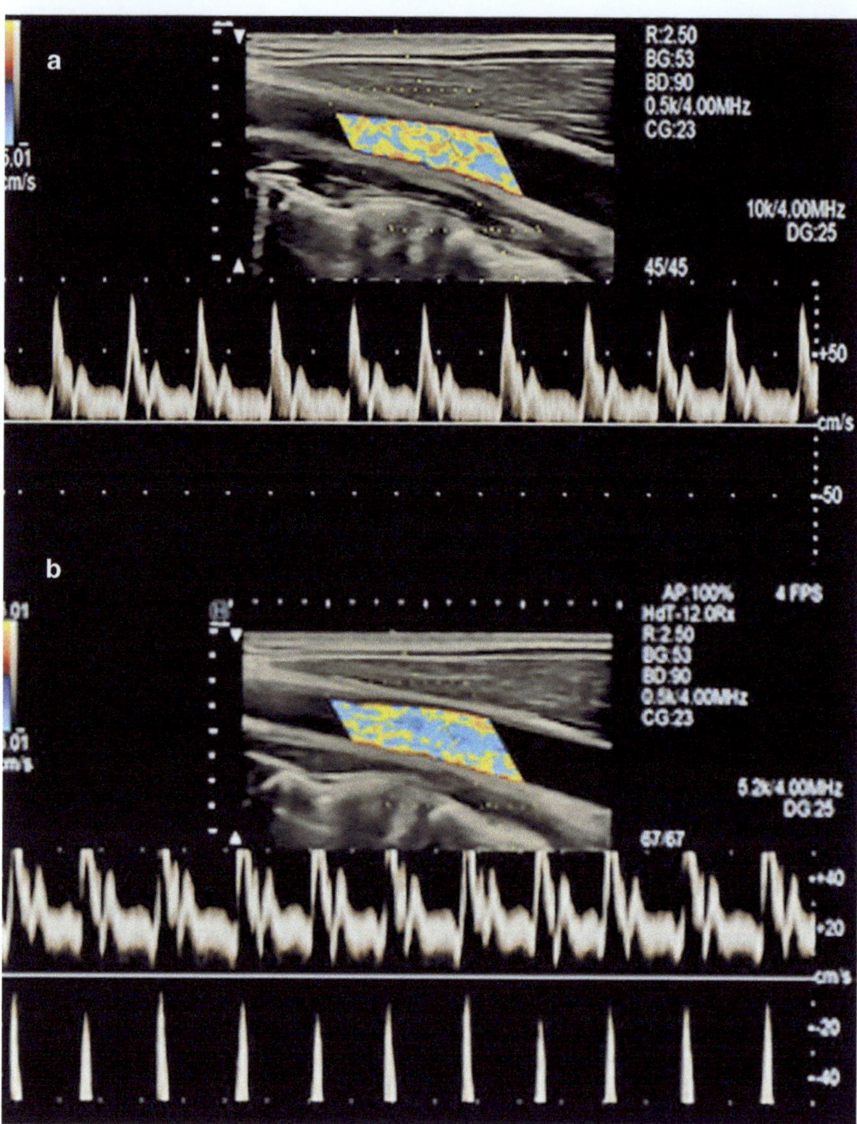

Fig. 3.1 Pulse repetition frequency (PRF) of pulse wave Doppler (PWD) too low (**a**) and optimized (**b**). In both images, the PRF is set much too low with aliasing in both

3.3.1.4   Wall Filter

The vessel wall's pulsations and other disruptive movements are removed by the wall filter. However, because the associated signals are suppressed by the filter settings, slow blood flow components of the spectral curve (such as low-end diastolic

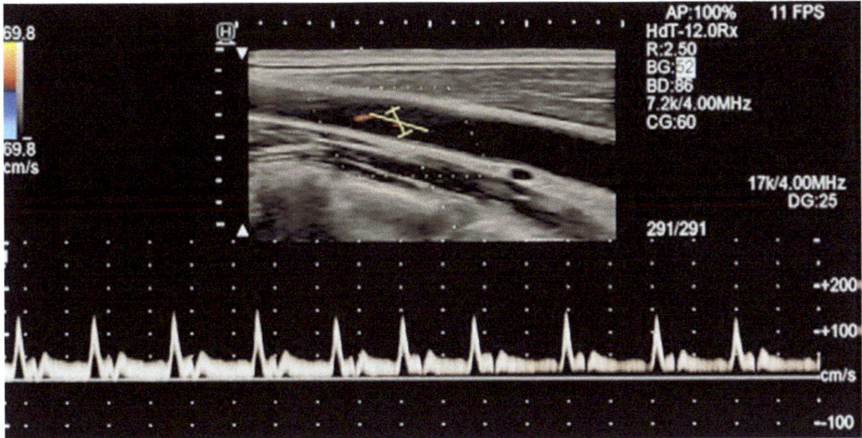

Fig. 3.2 The influence on the Doppler spectrum by enhanced wall filter settings. The filter blanks out signals corresponding to slower flow

velocities or a sluggish reverse flow) may not be visible. Thus, image optimization can improve the aesthetics but could also hide diagnostic information (Fig. 3.2). For penile Doppler examinations, we recommend turning off or adjusting the wall filter to a low setting.

3.3.1.5 Sweep Speed

The Doppler spectrum's scrolling speed can be changed by the sweep speed. More heart cycles are seen at a slower sweep speed, which is useful for illustrating some diseases (manly arrhythmias). However, speeding up the sweep results in fewer cycles with more thorough descriptions of each. Sweep speed may usually be changed after several heart cycles have been recorded; hence, it can be done after the image has been frozen ("post-processing"). For an accurate measurement of the cavernous arteries' blood flow, we recommend seeing at least five heart cycles on the screen.

3.3.1.6 Gate/Sample Volume

To display the whole range of potential speeds, the size of the gate (Doppler window) should be chosen. The optimal size would be at least two-thirds the vessel's diameter. For cavernous arteries, which have small calipers, the gate size must be as small as possible, despite the fact that it will eventually reach the whole diameter of the vessel.

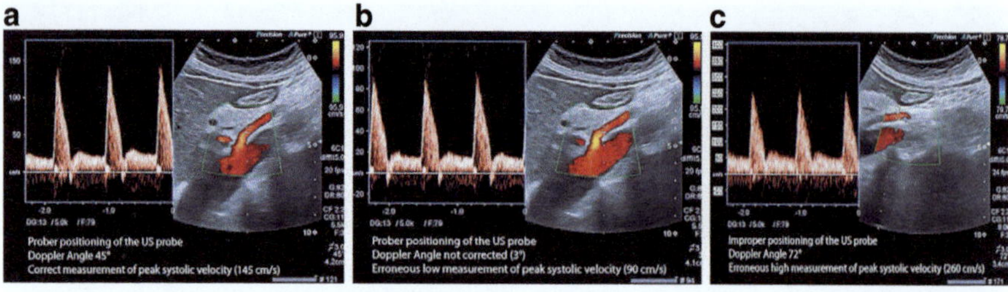

Fig. 3.3 Measurement of flow velocities in the superior mesenteric artery (SMA): following adjustment of scale to the velocity range typical for superior mesenteric artery (95.9 cm/s) and a correction of the Doppler angle to 45° correct measurement of the normal peak systolic velocity is possible: 145 cm/s (**a**); in case of no correction of Doppler angle, an erroneous low peak systolic velocity is measured (**b**; 90 cm/s); improper positioning of the US probe results in a Doppler angle of 72° (**c**), and correct measurement of flow velocity is impossible (erroneous measurement of a high peak systolic velocity in the range of mild stenosis)

3.3.1.7 Angle of Doppler

Using the appropriate rotary control or toggle switch, the Doppler angle must be adjusted to match the direction of the vessel. The Doppler angle needs to be adjusted between 0° and 60° (Fig. 3.3). Exact measurements are no longer attainable for Doppler angles greater than 60°. When an acceptable angle correction cannot be made, the US devices frequently utilize a marking to let the user know. When that occurs, the examiner should look for a position for the probe that allows a Doppler angle of 60° or less (i.e., penoscrotal junction normally has an optimal angle thanks to vertical anatomy of cavernous bodies). The user should know that angle corrections might be done by postprocessing on most US machines.

3.3.1.8 Inversion

The "Inversion" function swaps out the Doppler spectrum's mapping of the flow direction. Based on the flow towards or away from the probe, values are shown above or below the baseline.

3.3.1.9 Post-processing

To improve noise suppression during post-processing, the brightness of the image can be changed by altering the Doppler gain. The gain for arteries should be tuned so that it is easy to identify a frequency-free window. The color of the image and the angle correction can also be altered in post-processing. On more recent devices, the user can also change the baseline and sweep speed.

3.3.2   Automatically Optimizing Images

By altering the aforementioned parameters, the majority of high-end ultrasound machines can automatically adapt the Doppler settings. However, manual adjustments get the best image settings.

3.4   Color Doppler and Power Doppler Ultrasound

B-mode imaging and color-coding of flow information are integrated by color Doppler US (CD). PW frequently complements it. Therefore, CD is mostly utilized for focused vascular diagnostics.

There are two distinct modes. In the velocity mode, different colors (often red and blue) are used to represent the flow direction in reference to the transducer, and varying levels of color brightness and shading represent various flow velocities. The intensity mode, also known as Amplitude-Doppler or Power-Doppler, presents simply the flow presence without direction. This makes it possible to detect low-velocity blood flow with greater sensitivity, which could be eventually useful for cavernous arteries stenosis or subocclusions [5].

3.4.1   Parameters Settings in CD

When employing CD, the aforementioned crucial factors must be taken into account:

3.4.1.1   Transmission Frequency

It is possible to change the color Doppler frequency separately from the B-scan. Since penetration depth diminishes with frequency, a balance between acceptable penetration and sensitivity must be found. Due of the superficial nature of penile structures, high transmission frequencies should be preferably used.

3.4.1.2   Pulse Repetition Frequency/Scale

The displayed velocity range is determined by the PRF. When the scale's maximum flow velocity is reached, aliasing artifacts appear. Aliasing on CD could be indicative for stenosis if the set up is correctly placed as shown in Fig. 3.4 [6–8]. Low PRF values are utilized in micro-CD to reduce aliasing, while higher PRF levels are used in macro-CD to avoid false-negative vascularization results. In penile Doppler studies, we recommend setting the PRF to less than 5 cm/s

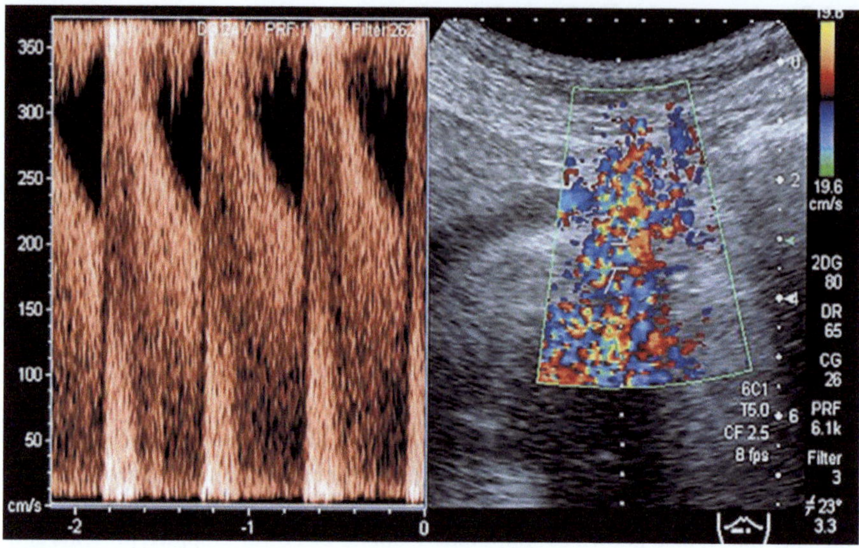

Fig. 3.4 Aliasing with CDUS and PWD in celiac trunk stenosis

3.4.1.3   Baseline

As the baseline is shifted up or down, the presentation of the flow velocity range changes. Baseline adjustment has no clinical benefit for CD.

3.4.1.4   Color Doppler Box

The box, where the flow is shown, ought to be adjusted according to the structure size requirements. The temporal resolution and frame rate are both improved by a reduced box size. Using the trackball, touchpad, and "set" button, the size and positioning of the box can be customized. Using linear array transducers, the examiner is able to steer the insonation angle. The retrieved flow information is better and more accurate the narrower the Doppler angle is between the transducer and the target vessel (Fig. 3.5).

3.4.1.5   Doppler Steering and Angle

An angle above 60° leads to incorrect flow velocities and cannot be corrected manually or technically; hence the Doppler angle must not be above this threshold which tends to impair the color representation of blood flow. Although steering the Doppler angle in the case of linear arrays is conceivable, it lessens the sensitivity of flow detection. Therefore, it is preferable to properly set the transducer in the beginning with the intention of obtaining a smaller Doppler angle between 0° and 30°.

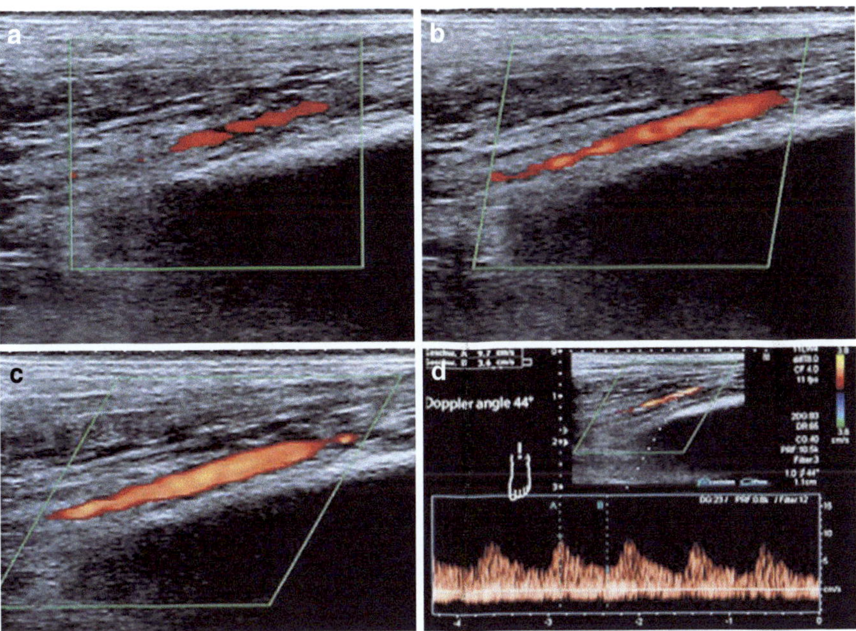

Fig. 3.5 Influence of beam steering on visualization of slow postocclusive flow in tibial artery. Scale was adjusted to low flow velocities (3.8 cm/s): no beam steering with poor visibility of flow (**a**). Beam steering (**b**: 15°; **c**: 30°) improves visibility and allows correct PWD measurement of the peak systolic velocity (9.7 cm/s) with an acceptable Doppler angle of 44° (**d**)

3.4.1.6   Inversion

By selecting "invert," you can switch the color spectrum. Since each color is chosen separately, the display's flow pattern should be understood using the color bar on the right or left side of the screen. By default, flow moving away from the transducer is shown as blue, while flow moving towards it is represented as red. Inversion can be useful for deliberately showing arteries in red and veins in blue, but if different providers are not familiar with the same inversion option, this could lead to confusion.

3.4.1.7   Gain

After initially increasing the color Doppler gain, it is recommended to gradually reduce it until the so-called "blooming" artifacts vanish (Fig. 3.6).

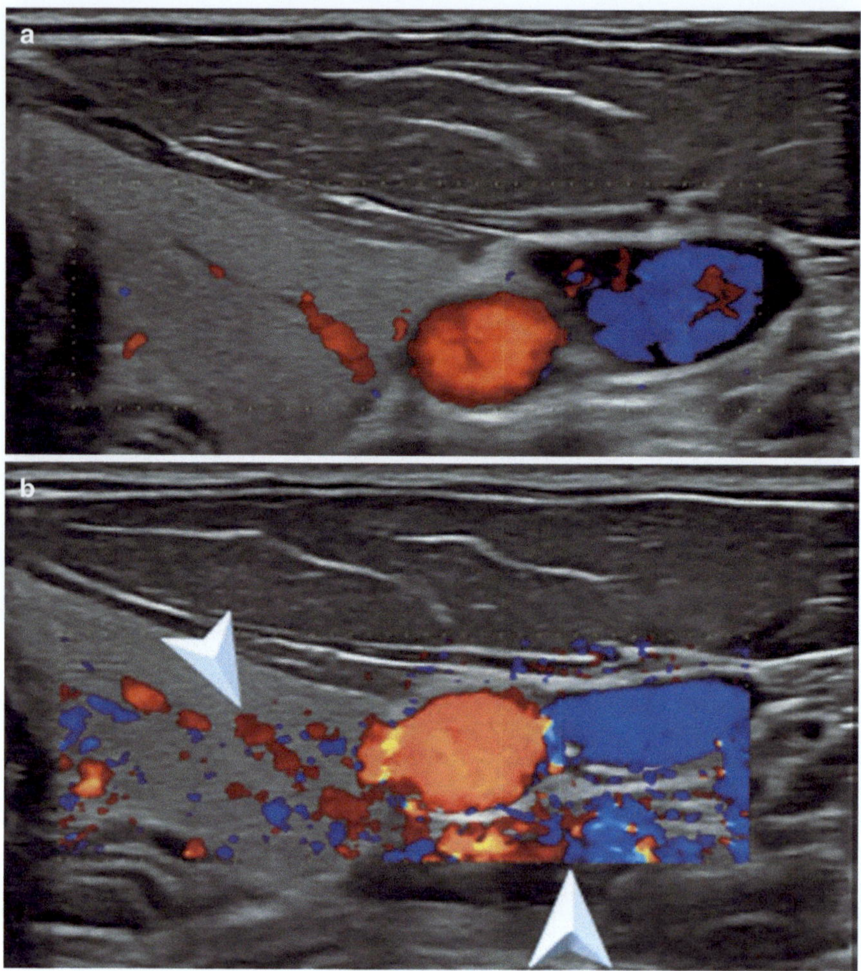

Fig. 3.6 Gain optimized (**a**), and too high with additional color artifacts, the so-called "blooming" phenomenon, around the actual vessels (arrows) (**b**)

3.5   Duplex and Triplex Modes

B-mode imaging can be combined with CD and PW. While "Duplex imaging" combines grayscale imaging with either CD or PW, "Triplex imaging" involves the examiner using all three modalities. By using CD to locate the target vessel initially, this technique can then be used to measure an additional flow by hitting the "Update" button. Here, the CD image is frozen and only PW is operating in real time. In Triplex mode, more recent devices can also simultaneously show B-scan, CD, and PW. However, examiners should be aware that Duplex mode is often preferred because using Triplex mode may decrease image quality and significantly slows frame rate.

3.6   Conclusion

This chapter provides an overview of information, techniques, and suggestions for spectral and color Doppler ultrasound parameter tuning to get the greatest image quality possible in penile Doppler evaluation. The most crucial variables are the following: transmission frequency, pulse repetition frequency (scale), baseline, wall filter, gain, sweep speed, sample volume, Doppler angle, inversion mode, post-processing parameters, automatic image optimization, size and angle steering of the color Doppler box, and the Duplex and Triplex modes.

References

1. Zander D, Hüske S, Hoffmann B, Cui X-W, Dong Y, Lim A, et al. Ultrasound image optimization ("knobology"): B-mode. Ultrasound Int Open. 2020;6(01):E14–24.
2. Atkinson NS, Bryant RV, Dong Y, Maaser C, Kucharzik T, Maconi G, et al. How to perform gastrointestinal ultrasound: anatomy and normal findings. World J Gastroenterol. 2017;23(38):6931.
3. El Haddad M, De Backer T, De Buyzere M, Devos D, Swillens A, Segers P, et al. Grading of mitral regurgitation based on intensity analysis of the continuous wave Doppler signal. Heart. 2017;103(3):190–7.
4. Jenssen C, Tuma J, Möller K, Cui X, Kinkel H, Uebel S, et al. Ultrasound artifacts and their diagnostic significance in internal medicine and gastroenterology-part 2: color and spectral Doppler artifacts. Zeitschrift fur Gastroenterologie. 2016;54(6):569–78.
5. Evans DH, Jensen JA, Nielsen MB. Ultrasonic colour Doppler imaging. Interface focus. 2011;1(4):490–502.
6. Dietrich C, Ignee A, Seitz K-H, Caspary W. Duplexsonographie der Viszeralarterien. Ultraschall Med. 2001;22(06):247–57.
7. Dietrich C, Jedrzejczyk M, Ignee A. Sonographic assessment of splanchnic arteries and the bowel wall. Eur J Radiol. 2007;64(2):202–12.
8. Ignee A, Boerner N, Bruening A, Dirks K, von Herbay A, Jenssen C, et al. Duplexsonography of the mesenteric vessels—a critical evaluation of inter observer variability. Z Gastroenterol. 2016;54(04):304–11.

Chapter 4
Penile Anatomy and Physiology of Erection

4.1 Introduction

The penis is the main anatomical structure for the purpose of performing a medical specialized evaluation of the male erectile function. It is located in the urogenital triangle, between the perineal membrane above and the deep perineal fascia below. It is a complex structure with many different anatomic details that should be of great interest for those willing to perform penile ultrasound studies. In this chapter, we aimed at discussing the most relevant aspects that a proficient examiner should master.

4.2 Anatomy

4.2.1 Penile Anatomical Structures

The penis is made up of three main parts: the glans, shaft, and crura. When referring to the anatomical position of the penis, the dorsal aspect is facing towards the head and the ventral side towards the feet. The dorsal portion of the penis consists of two parallel corporal bodies, while the ventral aspect contains the corpus spongiosum, which encloses the urethra. The corpora cavernosa is surrounded by the tunica albuginea, while the Buck's fascia or the deep fascia of the penis is a continuation of the deep perineal fascia that encases both the corpora cavernosa and corpus spongiosum. Although an intercavernosal septum of the penis separates the corpora cavernosa internally, this structure is not continuous and allows a wide communication between both corpora. The finding of a complete penile corporal septum leading to isolated corporal bodies a rare malformation in which the corpora cavernosa are completely isolated and function independently and might lead to lateral deformity,

© The Author(s), under exclusive license to Springer Nature
Switzerland AG 2024
E. d. P. Miranda, F. Carneiro, *Penile Color Duplex-Doppler Ultrasound in
Erectile Dysfunction Diagnosis and Management*,
https://doi.org/10.1007/978-3-031-55649-4_4

hinge defect of the shaft, poor response to PDE5i, and unilateral erection following intracavernous injection of vasoactive agents [1].

The most proximal part of the penis comprises the bulb, crura, and ischiocavernosus and bulbospongiosus muscles. The crura of the penis lie laterally between the two corpora cavernosa in the median plane. The penile suspensory ligament (PSL) attaches the symphysis pubis, and the tunica albuginea in the midline serves to provide support to the erect penis to maintain a suitable angle during sexual intercourse. The PSL is one part of the suspensory apparatus of the penis, which includes the fundiform and subarcuate ligaments. In addition, the PSL sends fibers that surround the deep dorsal vein of the penis, potentially playing a role in the veno-occlusive mechanism of erection when the erect penis is pressed against the pubis. Although the PSL is a physiologic structure that is usually not evaluated in penile hemodynamic studies with Doppler ultrasound, some patients may complain of penile deformities following abnormal penile angles as a result of PSL conditions. Traumatic or surgical damage to the PSL ligamentous structures can lead to a change in the erectile angle, marked instability, pain, and a rotational deformity occasionally. Young patients with excessive congenital fixation of the PSL may have the penis excessively close to the lower abdomen, mimicking a dorsal curvature [2].

The glans penis is the distal part of the penis, and its proximal portion is called the corona, separated from the body of the penis by the neck of the corona glans. The meatus, the opening to the urethra, is located at the tip of the glans. Loose connective tissue is present between the thin skin of the penis and the tunica albuginea. The prepuce or foreskin is a second skin layer covering the glans penis, with the frenulum of the prepuce connecting it to the urethral surface of the penis glans [3].

4.2.2 Tunica Albuginea

The tunica is a multilayered structure that provides both flexibility and rigidity to the penis. Studies using cadaveric microscopy have revealed that the tunica consists of an irregular lattice of elastic fibers on a collagen framework. Anatomical and mechanical characteristics of the tunica albuginea are definitely a critical component for an adequate penile rigidity [4].

The tunica albuginea consists basically of two primary layers: an inner circular layer that encases and supports the erectile tissue found within the corpora cavernosa and corpus spongiosum and an outer longitudinal layer that covers only the corpora cavernosa. This outer layer extends from the glans penis to the proximal crura. Classic anatomical studies revealed the existence of intracavernous pillars, which extend from the inner tunica at approximately the 2 and 10 o'clock positions to the ventral intercorporal septum. It is believed that these pillars enhance the

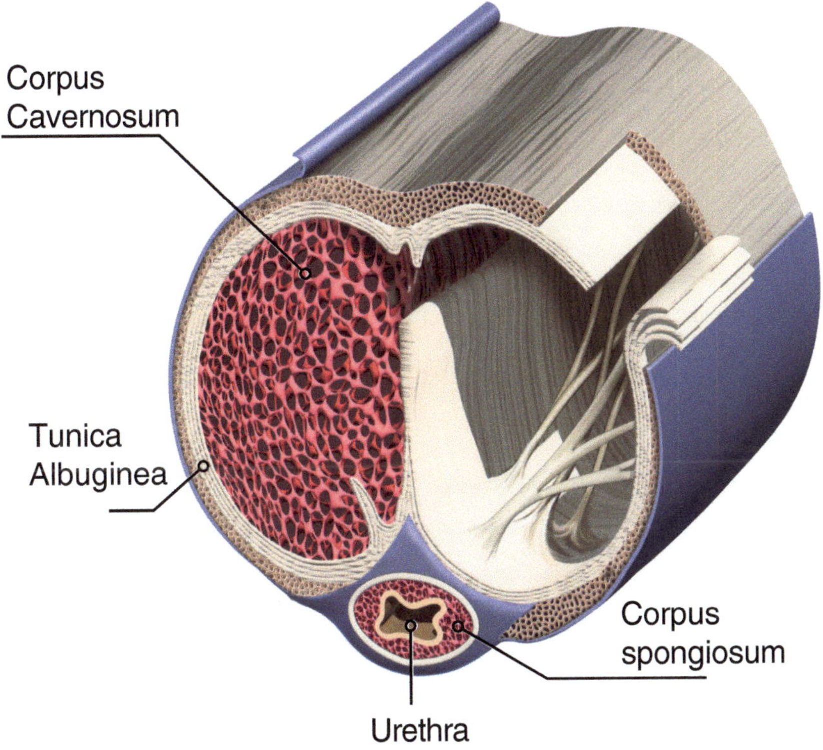

Fig. 4.1 Anatomical representation of the tunica albuginea

septum's structural integrity and provide critical geometric support to the erectile tissue, as demonstrated in Fig. 4.1 [5]. The intracavernous pillars are believed to strengthen the septum and provide crucial geometric support to the erectile tissue. Moreover, the pillars became more prominent and larger within the distal corpus cavernosum. This additional support structure could help the penis resist buckling forces and maintain distal stability during intercourse.

4.2.3 Arterial Supply

The superficial arterial irrigation of the penis is mainly supplied by the superficial external pudendal arteries, which are branches from the femoral artery. However, the internal pudendal arteries' branches are the primary source of blood supply for the penis to maintain a normal erectile function. The terminal branch of the internal pudendal artery is known as common penile artery that subdivides into three main branches as shown in Fig. 4.2:

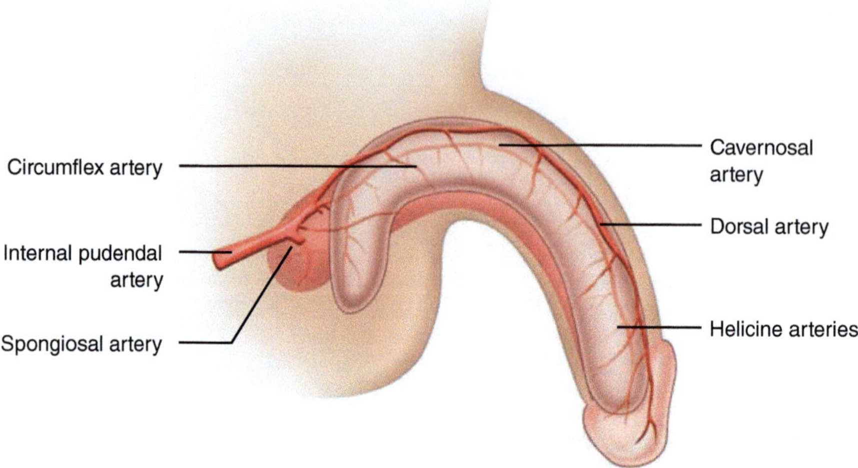

Fig. 4.2 Most commonly described arterial supply to the penis and main branches

1. The bulbourethral artery, also known as spongiosal artery, is usually the first branch directed to the penis. It passes through the deep penile (Buck's) fascia to supply the bulbous part of the corpus spongiosum, urethra, and bulbourethral gland.
2. The dorsal artery runs along the dorsum of the penis in each side, between the dorsal nerve and deep dorsal vein. It gives off circumflex branches that accompany the circumflex veins, with the terminal branches being located in the glans penis. The dorsal artery enters the penile shaft as the terminus of the internal pudendal artery.
3. The cavernosal artery, also known as the deep penile artery, is usually a single artery that arises on each side and enters the corpus cavernosum at the crus. The cavernosal arteries usually run through the center of each corpora cavernosa to supply the erectile tissue, giving off the helicine arteries, which play an integral role during an erection. This is the single most important vessel in penile hemodynamic studies, since Doppler parameters are usually assessed in the most proximal aspect of the dominant artery just after reaching the corporal bodies. Here it is important to recognize potential anatomic variations, which are seen in up to 40% of cases [6, 7]. Some common variations are extrapenile bifurcations with two or more dominant cavernosal arteries, dorso-cavernosal perforators, and intercavernosal branches. Patients with arterial insufficiency due to atherosclerosis may develop collateral circulation within the penis in order to maintain adequate blood flow during an erection. In such case, unusual dominant arteries may be seen.

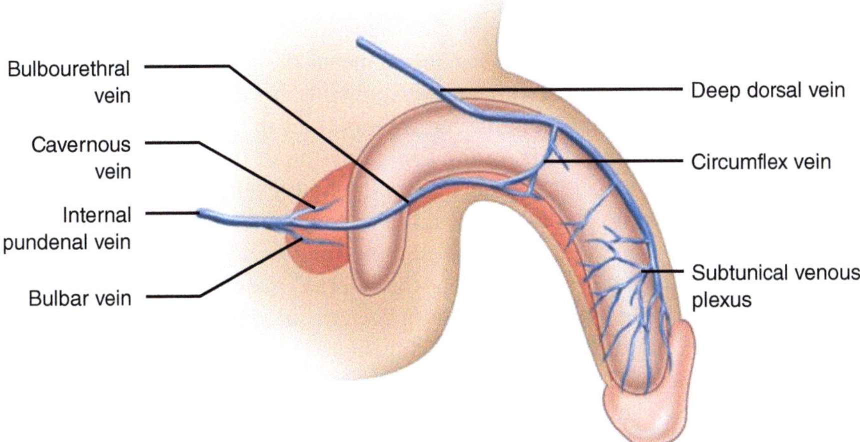

Fig. 4.3 Schematic drawing of penile venous drainage. Superficial and deep veins and subtunical venous plexus related to the mechanism of veno-occlusion. (TRANSLATION: veia pudenda interna—internal pudendal vein; veia bulbar—bulbar vein; veia cavernosa—cavernous vein; veia bulbouretral—bulbourethral vein; veia dorsal profunda—deep dorsal vein; veia circunflexa—circumflex vein, plexo venoso subtunical—subtunical venous plexus)

4.2.4 Venous Outflow

The venous drainage of the penis is traditionally divided into venous systems: the superficial, intermediate, and deep. The outline of penile venous outflow is demonstrated in Fig. 4.3.

The dartos fascia located on the upper side of the penis houses multiple superficial veins that converge at the base, forming a single superficial dorsal vein. Generally, this vein drains into the great saphenous veins through the superficial external pudendal veins. Many patients complain of the unusual appearance that these veins might acquire. Fact is that these veins are very numerous and might have different conformations throughout the years without any compromise to the erectile mechanism.

The intermediate system, which is situated beneath Buck's fascia, consists of the deep dorsal and circumflex veins. The deep dorsal vein is situated in the central groove between the two corpora cavernosa and is created by 5–8 veins originating from the glans penis, forming the retrocoronal plexus. On the lateral side of the cavernosa, the circumflex veins form a ring-shaped structure that runs underneath the dorsal arteries and nerves. These veins ultimately drain into the deep dorsal vein, and they receive blood from both the emissary and circumflex veins. The deep dorsal vein then runs below the symphysis pubis at the same level as the suspensory ligament, and it exits the shaft of the penis at the crus, draining into the prostatic plexus. It is important to make a distinction between the superficial and deep dorsal vein of the penis. The deep dorsal vein receives blood from the venous plexus, which receives drained blood from the cavernous spaces, while the superficial dorsal vein drains blood from the skin and subcutaneous tissue of the penis.

The crural and cavernosal veins are responsible for the deep venous drainage. The crural veins arise from the midline, in the gap between the crura. The cavernosal veins are formed from the consolidation of the emissary veins and unite to create a significant venous channel, which eventually drains into the internal pudendal vein. Additionally, three to four small cavernosal veins run laterally between the corpus spongiosum and the penis's crus for a length of 2–3 cm before ultimately draining into the internal pudendal veins.

Abnormalities in the venous system have been traditionally implicated in generating some types of vascular erectile dysfunction. Therefore, some authors have advocated that surgery or procedures that might increase the pressure in the penile venous system would eventually improve erection rigidity. However, it is important to highlight that that there are ultimately four sources of venous drainage from the corporal bodies: dorsal veins, spongiosal veins, cavernosal veins, and crural veins. These compressive procedures cannot restrict outflow from cavernosal or crural veins entirely, which will generally lead to minimal gain in erectile rigidity [8].

4.2.5   Nerve Supply

The nerves to the penis are derived from the pudendal and cavernous nerves. The nerve supply to the erectile tissue is provided by the cavernous nerves, which consist of a mixture of parasympathetic and visceral afferent fibers. The cavernous nerves have an intrinsic anatomic relation with the prostatic capsule and run in the crus and corpora of the penis, primarily dorsomedial to the cavernosal arteries. That is one of the reasons why there is a high prevalence of erectile dysfunction following radical prostatectomy. In order to remove the whole gland, the surgeon has to perform a dissection of the prostate capsule from the nerve fibers, which will eventually lead to temporary or permanent damage to parasympathetic innervation of the penis.

The pudendal nerves supply somatic motor and sensory innervation to the penis. The dorsal nerve of penis is one of the terminal branches of the pudendal nerve. Soon after entering the shaft; it gives off branches that will diverge to supply the ventral aspect of the penis and continues its dorsal course to reach the distal shaft and glans. Regional blockage of the dorsal nerve of the penis using local anesthetics will allow for in-office surgical manipulation of the penis. A summary of the penile nerve supply is shown in Fig. 4.4.

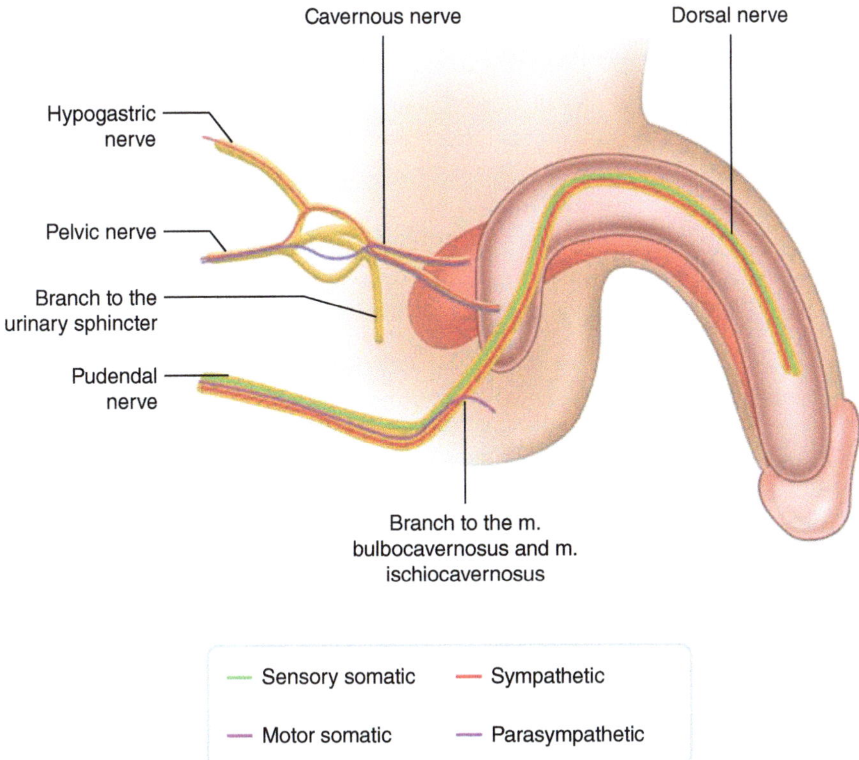

Fig. 4.4 Penile innervation related to erection depicting the main autonomic and sensory neuronal pathways. (TRANSLATION: nervohipogástrico—hypogastric nerve; nervopélvico—pelvic nerve, nervo pudenda—pudendal nerve; ramo para o m. bulbocavernosos e m. isquiocavernosos—branch to the m. bulbocavernosus and m. ischiocavernosus; ramo para o esfíncterurinário—branch to the urinary sphincter; nervocavernoso—cavernous nerve; nervo dorsal—dorsal nerve; somático sensorial—sensory somatic; somático motor—motor somatic; simpatico—sympathetic; parassimpático—parasympathetic)

4.3 Physiology of Erection

From a biological standpoint, an erection is a complex process that involves the proper functioning of multiple systems and organs. Essentially, penile erection and detumescence are hemodynamic phenomena controlled by neural stimuli, with cavernous smooth muscle playing an important role.

During sexual stimulation, nerve impulses cause the release of neurotransmitters from the cavernous nerve terminals and relaxing factors from the penile endothelial cells, resulting in relaxation of the smooth muscle in the arteries and arterioles that supply the erectile tissue and, consequently, a considerable increase in penile blood flow. At the same time, relaxation of the trabecular smooth muscle increases the compliance of the sinuses, facilitating rapid filling and expansion of the sinusoidal system. The subtunical venous plexuses are therefore compressed between the trabeculae and the tunica albuginea, resulting in near-total venous occlusion, with an intracavernous pressure of approximately 100 mmHg in the complete erection phase.

4.3.1 Autonomic Central Nervous System and Peripheric Control

Stimulation of the cerebral cortex through the senses of smell, sight, sound, and touch promotes activation of the parasympathetic pathways that promote erection. The autonomic pathways descend through the spinal cord to the peripheral autonomic nerves through the hypogastric plexus and cavernous nerve bundles to the erectile tissue. Animal studies have identified the medial preoptic area and the paraventricular nucleus of the hypothalamus and hippocampus as important centers for the integration of sexual function and penile erection. Parasympathetic stimulation leads to the release of nitric oxide by non-adrenergic, non-cholinergic nerve endings that reach the penis. Nitric oxide is considered the primary neurotransmitter responsible for the relaxation of erectile tissue. The pudendal nerve mainly carries sensory input, which is part of the penile reflex arc that also assists in the smooth muscle relaxation of the cavernous tissue [9].

4.3.2 Blood Flow and Veno-Occlusive Mechanism

The erectile tissue is mainly composed of smooth muscle, elastic fibers, and endothelium, which together form the sinusoids of corpora cavernosa. As explained earlier in this chapter, arterial supply is achieved through the internal pudendal artery, which branches out and gives origin to the cavernous artery and to the helicine arteries. The venous drainage of the cavernous tissue is performed by a surface and deep vein system; however, the subtunical venules promote blood exit from the intracavernous space during erection. During the flaccid state, the erectile tissue is predominantly stimulated by sympathetic fibers with dominant adrenergic output that induce contraction of the smooth muscle and maintain low intracavernous pressures. However, blood flow grows by the order of 5–6 times during sexual stimulus without changes in the systemic blood pressure. The smooth muscle relaxes and expands, as the sinusoids get full of blood. This expansion generates relative venous drainage reduction, mainly because of the passive venoconstriction of subtunical veins, which triggers the veno-occlusive mechanism and allows axial rigidity to increase exponentially when the compression of subtunical venules is complete, as demonstrated in Fig. 4.5 [10].

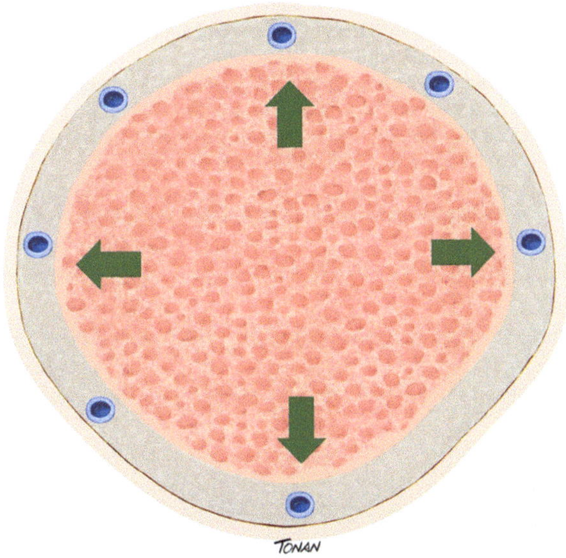

Fig. 4.5 Illustrative demonstration of the veno-occlusive mechanism through the compressive forces of the erectile tissue at subtunical venules

4.4 Conclusions

A thorough understanding of the main principles involved in penile anatomy and physiology is of great importance for those who provide care for men with sexual and erectile dysfunction. This review contains knowledge that is required for the correct execution of penile hemodynamic studies through Doppler ultrasound, since identification of anatomical structures is essential during the examination. Moreover, understanding the nuances of the erectile physiology is required for the correct interpretation of the results.

References

1. Henriquez KI, Brock G. Case: primary erectile dysfunction due to congenital isolated cavernous bodies. Can Urol Assoc J. 2017;11(9):E385–E7.
2. Ralph O, Shroff N, Anfosso M, Blecher G, Ralph D. Repair of the penile suspensory ligament for congenital and acquired pathology. BJU Int. 2019;124(4):687–92.
3. Tu LH, Spektor M, Ferrante M, Mathur M. MRI of the penis: indications, anatomy, and pathology. Curr Probl Diagn Radiol. 2020;49(1):54–63.
4. Pagano MJ, Weinberg AC, Deibert CM, Hernandez K, Alukal J, Zhao L, et al. Penile intracavernosal pillars: lessons from anatomy and potential implications for penile prosthesis placement. Int J Impot Res. 2016;28(3):114–9.
5. Brock G, Hsu GL, Nunes L, von Heyden B, Lue TF. The anatomy of the tunica albuginea in the normal penis and Peyronie's disease. J Urol. 1997;157(1):276–81.
6. Erdoğru T, Kaplancan T, Aker O, Aras N. Cavernosal arterial anatomic variations and its effect on penile hemodynamic status. Eur J Ultrasound. 2001;14(2–3):141–8.

7. Sakamoto H, Nagata M, Saito K, Okumura T, Yoshida H. Anatomic variations of cavernous arteries and their effect on measurement of hemodynamic parameters: a power Doppler study. Urology. 2004;63(3):539–44.
8. Miranda EP, Taniguchi H, Cao DL, Hald GM, Jannini EA, Mulhall JP. Application of sex aids in men with sexual dysfunction: a review. J Sex Med. 2019;16(6):767–80.
9. Dean RC, Lue TF. Physiology of penile erection and pathophysiology of erectile dysfunction. Urol Clin N Am. 2005;32(4):379–95.
10. Meldrum DR, Burnett AL, Dorey G, Esposito K, Ignarro LJ. Erectile hydraulics: maximizing inflow while minimizing outflow. J Sex Med. 2014;11(5):1208–20.

Chapter 5
Clinical Aspects of Erectile Dysfunction

5.1   Introduction

Many professionals who perform penile Doppler ultrasound (PDU) examinations around the world are radiologists or other medical professionals not necessarily trained in the management of patients with erectile dysfunction (ED). Although this is not a requirement per se, it is the authors' understanding that PDU examiners should have a distinct understanding of the most relevant clinical aspects of ED. Being aware of the clinical pathways and eventual implications of abnormal hemodynamic parameters found in these examinations will improve the overall quality of PDU. This chapter consists of a practical review of the most relevant and up-to-date concepts regarding the evaluation, diagnosis, and management of ED.

5.2   Definition

Erectile dysfunction (ED) is defined as the consistent inability to attain or maintain an erection sufficient for satisfactory sexual intercourse. The term impotence has traditionally been used for centuries and is still used in lay terms. However, it has been replaced by ED since 1992 and should not be used in clinical practice because it generates confusion and has been considered pejorative [1].

5.3   Epidemiology

ED is a very prevalent condition, being present in 20–45% of the general population and up to 60% of men aged 65–85 [2]. Although ED is commonly associated with older men, recent studies have shown that a significant proportion of younger men

© The Author(s), under exclusive license to Springer Nature
Switzerland AG 2024
E. d. P. Miranda, F. Carneiro, *Penile Color Duplex-Doppler Ultrasound in
Erectile Dysfunction Diagnosis and Management*,
https://doi.org/10.1007/978-3-031-55649-4_5

are also affected. In fact, research has found that one in four men seeking medical help for ED are under the age of 40 [3].

The impact of ED on both the patient and their partner's quality of life and sexual satisfaction can be significant. Unfortunately, studies have also suggested 11.6–34.4% will ever seek medical help for their condition [4]. This represents both a gap in medical care for men's health and an opportunity for professionals who might occupy this niche and provide such care.

5.4   Etiology (Psychogenic vs. Organic)

Previously, it was believed that erectile dysfunction (ED) was caused by either psychological or physiological factors. However, it is now recognized that ED is a complex condition with multiple factors involved, and its management requires a biopsychosocial approach [5].

ED is most commonly classified as psychogenic, organic, or mixed etiology. Organic ED encompasses neurogenic, endocrinologic, vasculogenic, medication-induced, anatomic, or trauma related [6]. Risk factors for cardiovascular disease such as hypertension, diabetes, smoking, obesity, and dyslipidemia are also well-established risk factors for ED [7].

On the other hand, ED that is not caused by an organic condition is also referred to as psychogenic or adrenaline-mediated ED. While it has not been extensively researched, it is a crucial aspect to consider when diagnosing and treating men with this condition. Psychogenic ED is often associated with stress, depression, and anxiety, which manifest through increased nervousness about one's ability to perform during sexual activity. This connection comes as no surprise, considering that noradrenaline, the primary neurotransmitter responsible for suppressing erections, is involved.

Moreover, it is also very important to evaluate the situational and relationship factors in men with ED even in those with known organic ED. It is a known fact that the quality of a couple's relationship plays a pivotal role in determining the success of their sexual activity. Any sexual dysfunction experienced by one partner can have a significant impact on the entire couple, leading to distress, relationship issues, and even worsening of the initial sexual problem. In other words, all sexual dysfunctions, including those with well-established organic causes like post prostatectomy ED, can be stressful and lead to psychological disturbances [6]. It is the authors understanding that every patient with ED has a certain degree of a psychogenic component, and PDU examiners must always be aware of this phenomenon. However, there are some clinical hints during evaluation of ED that might indicate the predominant component, as indicated in Table 5.1.

There are multiple described mechanisms that might lead to organic ED. Table 5.2 displays a list of potential causes of ED according to different etiology categories. Vasculogenic ED is recognized as the most common cause of organic erectile

Table 5.1 Differentiating aspect of psychogenic vs. organic ED

Psychogenic	Organic
Sudden onset	Gradual onset
Intermittent function (variability, situational)	Often progressive
Loss of sustaining capability	Consistently poor response
Excellent nocturnal erection	Erection better in standing position than lying down (in the presence of venous leak)
Response to phosphodiesterase type 5 inhibitors is likely to be excellent	

Adapted from Yafi et al.

Table 5.2 ED categories and associated risk factors

Category	Risk factors
Vasculogenic arterial	Macroangiopathy or microangiopathy (e.g., atherosclerosis, vasculitis, trauma, etc.)
Venogenic dysfunction	Venoocclusive mechanism dysfunction
Sinusoidal	Penile collagenization; penile fibrosis
Neurogenic	Degenerative disorders (multiple sclerosis or Parkinson disease), stroke, CNS tumors, and spinal cord injury, post prostatectomy
Hormonal	Hypogonadism, hyperprolactinemia, hyperthyroidism, hypothyroidism, Cushing disease, panhypopituitarism
Anatomic or structural	Peyronie disease, penile fracture, hypospadias, epispadias, or micropenis
Psychogenic	Depression, anxiety, stress, or partner-related issues
Drug induced	Antihypertensive agents, antidepressants, antipsychotic agents, antiandrogens, recreational drugs (alcohol, heroin, marijuana)

dysfunction, and it can be an indication of an underlying vascular disorder, which can be a result of reduced blood flow, arterial insufficiency, or arterial stenosis resulting from vascular disease and endothelial dysfunction [6].

5.5 Clinical Evaluation

Performing a basic ED evaluation is fundamental to adequate exam conduction. Medical history, including comorbidities, medication use, and previous pelvic or retroperitoneal surgery must be questioned. The patient must be asked about his hardest erection in the bedroom scenario, which would be the minimal erection hardness to be obtained during the exam. This parameter is also known as BQE ("best quality erection" or "bedroom quality erection") and is very important to be observed during PDU examinations. Information about ED chronology and the permanence of nocturnal erections are quickly collected through straight questions and should not be forgotten.

5.5.1 Medical History

Regardless of the initial presenting symptom, patient evaluation always begins with obtaining a medical history. For patients who present with sexual dysfunction, a detailed sexual history is crucial in identifying the nature of the problem, potential biological and psychological factors, and any other contributing issues that may be relevant. In order to avoid discomfort for the patient, it is crucial to ask questions in a sensitive and respectful manner. It is also an important moment to inquire about sexual orientation and preferred sexual practices to have a better understanding of the patient's global perspective.

Other essential components of a full medical history include patient demographics, lifestyle and cultural beliefs, medical/psychological comorbidities, surgical history, medication history, and history of recreational substance use. Numerous comorbidities and lifestyle attributes are associated with increased risk for ED, including increasing age, diabetes, depression, cardiovascular disease, smoking, and lower urinary tract symptoms. Capturing these factors during medical history evaluation is essential [8].

Structured interviews and self-reported questionnaires can be helpful for clinicians of all experience levels in evaluating sexual health and related conditions. These tools consist of standardized questions that evaluate specific outcomes responses and might aid in facilitate better patient–physician relationships and minimize misunderstandings. Structured questionnaires are usually helpful in establishing the diagnosis of ED and classify patients according to disease severity. Several instruments have been published and are further discussed in other chapters of this book.

5.5.2 Physical Examination

To assess men with erectile dysfunction, a comprehensive physical examination should be conducted, including general and genital exam. A comprehensive general exam should include the evaluation of the chest to assess signs of gynecomastia (enlargement of the breasts) and body hair distribution, which might be signs of hypogonadism. Blood pressure, waist circumference, and body mass index should also be measured.

During genital examination, healthcare professionals have a chance to detect physical manifestations linked to erectile dysfunction. The evaluation of the penis in the flaccid condition can show the presence of Peyronie's disease, phimosis, or frenulum breve, which can contribute to erectile dysfunction. It is essential for the clinician to explain the medical necessity of the examination and seek the patient's permission beforehand, as some individuals may feel uncomfortable with a genital examination. Penile length measurements should be ideally performed at this time in the flaccid state, since it is a common source of complaints and the obtained measures might be used for patient counseling and reassurance. Physical examination might also help in identifying eventual difficulties for intracavernous injections during PDU.

The prostate and testes should also be examined. Small testes and/or a small prostate volume, in relation to the patient's age, may also indicate underlying hypogonadism.

5.6   Complementary Testing

The basic work-up of patients seeking medical care for ED needs to include a basic hormonal and biochemical tests. Among them, cholesterol, triglycerides, fasting glucose, and HbA1c levels are essential for evaluating cardiovascular and metabolic risks. To rule out hypogonadism, total testosterone and sex hormone-binding globulin are typically sufficient, while prolactin and thyroid hormone evaluation are limited to specific patients. If total or calculated free testosterone levels are low, prolactin and gonadotropin levels can help identify whether the problem is centrally or peripherally sourced.

In primary care settings, for most men with ED, additional diagnostic tests may be required if abnormal biochemical or hormonal values are detected (considered as second-line evaluation). To exclude overt diabetes mellitus, an oral glucose tolerance test is useful when fasting plasma glucose level is between $100–126$ mg dL^{-1} or HbA1c is $>5.7\%$. Furthermore, the need for further cardiovascular evaluation should be determined based on the criteria established by the Princeton III Consensus Panel [9].

5.7   Treatment Algorithms for ED

A new paradigm has emerged in the most recent ED guidelines, which suggests that shared decision-making is the cornerstone of the treatment and management of ED, a model that relies on the concepts of autonomy and respect for persons in the clinical encounter. It is also a process in which the patient and the clinician together determine the best course of therapy based on a discussion of the risks, benefits, and desired outcome. Using this approach, all men should be informed of all treatment options that are not medically contraindicated to determine the appropriate treatment. The clinician's role is to ensure that the man and his partner have a full understanding of the benefits and risks/burdens of the various management strategies [10].

Lifestyle modifications are usually recommended for men with ED since a positive impact of such strategy has been extensively demonstrated. PDE5 inhibitors are very effective and have a favorable safety profile, making them a valuable option as an initial pharmacotherapy for the vast majority of patients. Vacuum erection devices, intraurethral suppository, and intracavernosal injections with vasoactive substances are possibilities that might also be offered to patients, especially those with poor response or contraindications to PDE5 inhibitors. Surgical intervention with penile implants is usually a definitive treatment for severe and refractory, and patients should be well informed about the risk and benefits of this treatment modality.

5.8   Conclusions

Although PDU examination is not considered a medical consultation per se, it is very important for examiners to have a superior comprehension of the most relevant clinical aspects of ED, which is a multifaceted and prevalent condition that significantly impacts the quality of life for affected individuals. It is important to keep in mind that multiple etiological factors are usually contributing to the development of ED and that the distinction between organic vs. psychogenic ED is not always clear. Medical history, physical examination, and assessment biochemical and hormonal parameters are integral parts of a complete medical evaluation. However, the crucial role of a strong doctor-patient relationship, emphasizing the importance of a patient-centered approach in addressing individual concerns and preferences, should not be overlooked.

The medical knowledge from this chapter is a requirement for those willing to enhance their understanding of ED and develop tailored treatment strategies through PDU examinations. With a comprehensive understanding of the clinical aspects of ED, healthcare providers can offer personalized care and improve the overall quality of life and sexual health of their patients.

References

1. NIH. Impotence. NIH Consens Statement. 1992;10(4):1–33.
2. Gareri P, Castagna A, Francomano D, Cerminara G, De Fazio P. Erectile dysfunction in the elderly: an old widespread issue with novel treatment perspectives. Int J Endocrinol. 2014;2014:878670.
3. Capogrosso P, Colicchia M, Ventimiglia E, Castagna G, Clementi MC, Suardi N, et al. One patient out of four with newly diagnosed erectile dysfunction is a young man—worrisome picture from the everyday clinical practice. J Sex Med. 2013;10(7):1833–41.
4. Frederick LR, Cakir OO, Arora H, Helfand BT, McVary KT. Undertreatment of erectile dysfunction: claims analysis of 6.2 million patients. J Sex Med. 2014;11(10):2546–53.
5. Hatzichristou D, Kirana PS, Banner L, Althof SE, Lonnee-Hoffmann RA, Dennerstein L, et al. Diagnosing sexual dysfunction in men and women: sexual history taking and the role of symptom scales and questionnaires. J Sex Med. 2016;13(8):1166–82.
6. Yafi FA, Jenkins L, Albersen M, Corona G, Isidori AM, Goldfarb S, et al. Erectile dysfunction. Nat Rev Dis Prim. 2016;2:16003.
7. Voznesensky I, DeLay KJ, Hellstrom WJ. Advances in pharmacotherapy for erectile dysfunction and associated cardiac impact. Expert Opin Pharmacother. 2016;17(17):2281–9.

8. Mulhall JP, Giraldi A, Hackett G, Hellstrom WJG, Jannini EA, Rubio-Aurioles E, et al. The 2018 revision to the process of care model for evaluation of erectile dysfunction. J Sex Med. 2018;15(9):1280–92.
9. Nehra A, Jackson G, Miner M, Billups KL, Burnett AL, Buvat J, et al. The Princeton III consensus recommendations for the management of erectile dysfunction and cardiovascular disease. Mayo Clin Proc. 2012;87(8):766–78.
10. Burnett AL, Nehra A, Breau RH, Culkin DJ, Faraday MM, Hakim LS, et al. Erectile dysfunction: AUA guideline. J Urol. 2018;200(3):633–41.

Chapter 6
The Role of Penile Doppler Ultrasound in the Diagnosis and Management of Erectile Dysfunction

6.1 Introduction

The use of penile Doppler ultrasound (PDU) to evaluate erection dysfunction (ED) was first described by Lue et al. in 1985. PDU is often combined with intracavernosal injections (ICI) of vasoactive substances to test penile circulation under maximal pharmacological stimulation, offering insights into the functional aspects of an erection [1]. It is considered a noninvasive imaging technique used to examine the larger anatomical structure of the penis. PDU is also utilized in the assessment of Peyronie's disease (PD), as it allows the ability to characterize plaques and visualize calcification [2].

The traditional indications for penile ultrasound in urological practice include the evaluation of priapism, dorsal vein thrombosis, and penile tumors, which require the sole anatomic evaluation using B-mode ultrasound. However, most recent urological guidelines include the use of Doppler mode evaluation to enhance its diagnostic properties and allow for vascular evaluation of the penis.

6.2 Indications of Penile Doppler Ultrasound

Overall, PDU is a valuable and noninvasive tool in the evaluation of various conditions affecting male sexual health, particularly in the assessment of ED and penile vascular abnormalities. It provides critical information that helps clinicians make accurate diagnoses and formulate targeted treatment plans, ultimately improving patient outcomes and quality of life.

PDU is most indicated to evaluate young men with primary or secondary ED, in men with history of pelvic trauma or drug abuse, prior to surgical interventions for

© The Author(s), under exclusive license to Springer Nature Switzerland AG 2024
E. d. P. Miranda, F. Carneiro, *Penile Color Duplex-Doppler Ultrasound in Erectile Dysfunction Diagnosis and Management*,
https://doi.org/10.1007/978-3-031-55649-4_6

Table 6.1 Most relevant indications for performing PDU

Main indications for penile Doppler ultrasound studies
– Psychogenic ED
– Erectile function assessment in men with Peyronie's disease
– Failure to respond to PDE5i
– Assessment of cardiovascular risk
Secondary indications for penile Doppler ultrasound studies
– Post radical pelvic surgery (i.e., post radical prostatectomy ED)
– Medicolegal purposes

treating Peyronie's disease, to help in differentiating psychogenic vs. organic ED, and eventually in medicolegal cases [3]. It may also be helpful in identifying men with severe veno-occlusive dysfunction resulting in ED who are unlikely to respond to medical therapy and identify men who may be candidates for penile revascularization procedures. In the setting of PD, it is the most reliable tool to assess erectile function [4].

It is also important to mention that ED can be the first presenting symptom of multi-organ endothelial dysfunction. Certain comorbidities associated with one or more risk factors may require further hemodynamic investigation, and PDU may serve as a screening tool for that purpose. Some key indications for performing PDU are enumerated in Table 6.1. An in-depth analysis of each of these indications is elaborated in specific subsections of this chapter.

6.2.1   Psychogenic vs. Organic ED

There is a classic dichotomy in the evaluation of men with ED, which is trying to determine if one has psychogenic or organic ED. The diagnosis of organic ED occurs when there are disruptions in the arterial and/or venous blood flow to the penis or any other mechanism that are essential for sustaining a healthy erection. PDU plays a pivotal role in discerning whether the underlying cause of ED is organic or psychogenic in nature, as it facilitates the assessment of parameters like peak systolic velocity (PSV) and end-diastolic velocity (EDV), aiding in the differentiation between arterial insufficiency and veno-occlusive issues as the etiological factors.

Once organic causes of ED are ruled out, psychogenic causes of ED are usually considered. However, in most recent times, ED has been considered a multifactorial condition, and perhaps this differentiation is no longer crucial for the management of ED. In fact, it is the authors' understanding that most men with ED will have a certain degree of a psychogenic component that will require specialized care.

On the other hand, many patients with psychogenic ED are resistant to diagnosis and treatment and tend to believe that there should be any organic issue in their penile physiology. This is notably prevalent in younger individuals with ED, which might be also associated with depressive symptoms, pessimistic attitudes, and negative outlook on life. In such cases, PDU may be particularly helpful in ruling out organic causes of ED [5]. However, examiners must be careful because in older adult men with ED-linked comorbidities, components of psychogenic ED are also prevalent and might indicate a mixed etiology.

Moreover, interpreting low PSV measurements in men under the age of 30 with ED is crucial but requires careful consideration. Such findings might be a consequence of an increased sympathetic environment of a medical setting, the anxiety related to penile injections, and potential underlying psychological issues, as noted by the authors. These factors should always be considered when conducting PDU and emphasize the importance of high-quality examinations. Repeating PDU studies before contemplating further invasive diagnostic or therapeutic approaches may be an interesting option when in doubt.

6.2.2 ED Evaluation in Peyronie's Disease

Peyronie's disease is a combination of penile pain, fibrotic plaque formation, and penile curvature deformity, which can ultimately lead to ED. It has been demonstrated that PDU is effective in patients with PD and can guide appropriate therapeutic choices. The American Urological Association (AUA) recommends in-office erection test with or without PDU prior to invasive intervention for PD [6]. In this setting, PDU provides a hemodynamic study of penile blood flow and assessment of penile deformity, which can be particularly useful in cases with more extensive curvature and those with a history of ED, as it influences the decision-making process to select ideal candidates for grafting procedures.

Although guidelines support the use of validated questionnaires to quantify the severity of ED, this may be inadequate for men with PD when used alone [4]. Questionnaires such as the IIEF alone will most likely overestimate the severity of ED, since most men with PD will have a significant component of psychogenic ED or may have biomechanical instability secondary to severe penile deformity preventing adequate penetration ability. A recent study comparing PDU and IIEF in men with PD has revealed that abnormal vascular parameters were detected in only 45% of subjects, and even among men with severe ED, these vascular irregularities were observed in just 39% of the examinations [4]. These findings are relevant because guidelines medical recommend penile implants for men with PD and poor erectile function, which ideally should not be defined by anamnesis and ED questionnaires alone. Additional questionnaires such as the Peyronie's Disease Questionnaire (PDQ) may be instrumental in monitoring treatment progress for PD, but they do not comprehensively address the underlying ED. Therefore, the authors' understanding is that PDU is strongly recommended in this setting as it provides a comprehensive diagnostic approach for patients dealing with both PD and ED.

6.2.3   Non-responders to PDE5i

It is a fact that PDU may not benefit the management of all patients, and performing to every patient with ED is probably unnecessary. However, it does play an important role in specific populations experiencing ED because the ability to pinpoint the precise cause of non-response to PDE5i enables clinicians to tailor treatment strategies.

Phosphodiesterase type 5 inhibitors (PDE5i) constitute a cornerstone in the management of ED. However, a subset of patients, known as non-responders, do not experience the desired improvement in erectile function despite PDE5i therapy. PDU emerges as an indispensable tool in elucidating the underlying factors contributing to the lack of response and in optimizing therapeutic approaches.

Treatment with PDE5i is usually highly effective, reaching efficacy rates of about 85%. For an adequate PDE5i response, it is required an integrity in both neurological and vascular pathways. Therefore, an objective vascular testing with PDU that provides a physiologic diagnosis may help direct appropriate therapy because not all patients respond adequately to oral ED therapy [7]. In addition, the reasons behind this lack of response are often unclear as medical history, and standardized questionnaires may not capture structural abnormalities of the penis.

Therefore, we propose in terms of standardization purposes that PDU be administered in patients who do not respond to oral pharmacotherapy for ED. As these patients will likely need intracavernosal injections of vasoactive agents, PDU will also serve as a transition strategy from oral to ICI. PDU will eventually be able to demonstrate other anatomical abnormalities and the presence of subclinical PD [5].

6.2.4   Assessment of Cardiovascular Risk

PDU assesses the quality of arterial blood flow and sufficiency of veno-occlusive mechanisms, both necessary for an adequate erection. In other words, PDU provides a thorough overview of penile vascular health and gives a snapshot of overall vascular status. Arteriogenic ED represents a subtype of ED caused by penile arterial insufficiency and can represent an early manifestation of generalized vascular disease with risk factors paralleling those of cardiovascular disease.

Penile vasculature assessed during PDU can indicate cardiovascular disease and allow identification of men who are at the high risk of developing cardiovascular disease. Because the penile arteries measure 1–2 mm compared with the size of the coronary arteries (3–4 mm), clinically significant atherosclerosis and endothelial dysfunction may lead to earlier manifestation of disease in erectile tissue. Low PSVs together with cavernosal artery alterations usually indicate an arterial disease as the cause of ED. Moreover, the presence of calcifications involving the cavernosal artery on the B-mode survey scan can give clues to endothelial dysfunction, arterial insufficiency, and underlying atherosclerotic disease [8]. With advancements in the axial resolution of ultrasound probes, the evaluation of arterial wall thickness and plaque burden has become increasingly feasible and has emerged as a novel morphological parameter for the detection of atherosclerosis. Therefore, the physician evaluating ED has a unique opportunity to diagnose vascular impairment at a time when lifestyle changes and possible medical intervention have the potential to change morbidity and mortality of cardiovascular disease.

Cardiovascular disease is a major cause of morbidity and mortality in the USA, yet traditional risk factors can miss a significant population at risk for cardiac events. Thus, finding new predictors of cardiovascular disease risk may significantly decrease this burden and improve overall health. Recent studies have suggested that arteriogenic erectile dysfunction may be a nontraditional risk factor for cardiovascular disease and such diagnosis may provide a window of opportunity during which intervention can prevent or mitigate the development of cardiovascular disease [9]. This becomes evident in a study involving 49 men predominantly afflicted by arteriogenic erectile dysfunction (ED), all of whom had not undergone any previous cardiac assessments. Prior to undergoing stress echocardiography, penile Doppler ultrasound (PDU) was administered. Notably, 20% of the participants displayed anomalies on their stress echocardiograms, which encompassed severe cardiac wall motion irregularities—a notable contrast to the 2–3% incidence rate reported in the general population. Through both univariate and multivariate analyses, it was discerned that cavernosal artery insufficiency, delineated by PSV <30 cm/s, consistently emerged as a robust indicator for predicting an abnormal stress echocardiogram [10]. The important message is that ED is often a reentry point for men into health care after years of neglect.

6.3   Secondary Indication of PDU Studies

6.3.1   Post-radical Pelvic Surgery

Radical pelvic surgeries, such as radical prostatectomy, can have a significant impact on erectile function due to potential nerve damage and alterations in blood flow dynamics. PDU may be a valuable tool in assessing the vascular components contributing to ED post-radical pelvic surgery.

An underreported use of PDU is for men with ED following radical prostatectomy or cystectomy. PDU enables the evaluation of postoperative changes in penile blood flow. By measuring parameters like peak systolic velocity (PSV) and end-diastolic velocity (EDV), the vascular status of the penis can be accurately characterized. Changes in blood flow patterns can provide insights into potential vascular complications arising from surgery, aiding in the diagnosis and subsequent management of ED.

Nerve preservation during radical pelvic surgery is essential for maintaining erectile function. As an objective evaluation of postoperative cavernous nerve function is not available in clinical practice, assuring the vascular status and erectile tissue responsiveness may provide valuable information about long-term expectations of erectile function recovery. Moreover, PDU's noninvasive nature makes it a suitable tool for longitudinal monitoring of patients after radical pelvic surgery. This monitoring might aid in refining therapeutic approaches for managing post-surgical ED and enhancing patient satisfaction. A study evaluated 45 male patients with PDU who had a cystectomy, including 21 patients with nerve-sparing technique and 24 patients with non-nerve-sparing technique over the course of 12 months postoperatively. PSVs were comparable between the two groups during follow-up. EDV significantly deteriorated postoperatively compared to preoperative evaluation in both groups; however, gradual improvement in EDV was seen in the nerve-sparing group 12 months after surgery [11].

Although incorporating PDU into the evaluation of patients who have undergone radical pelvic surgery is not mandatory, it may offer valuable insights into the mechanisms underlying postoperative ED. For example, erectile function recovery usually takes up to 24 months to allow for nerve damage to fully recover. However, early detection of severe veno-occlusive dysfunction on PDU examination is usually irreversible and might unleash more invasive therapies without the need for unnecessary prolonged waiting intervals.

6.3.2 Medicolegal Cases

In cases where ED plays a role in legal matters such as divorce, rape, or personal injury claims, PDU can offer crucial insights. By assessing penile vascular function and identifying potential organic causes of ED, PDU assists in establishing a link between the alleged incident and the resulting ED. This objective data can serve as valuable evidence in legal proceedings. By aiding in establishing causation, offering a differential diagnosis, providing objective documentation, and impacting legal proceedings, PDU elevates the quality of evidence presented in the courtroom.

Moreover, by capturing real-time measurements of hemodynamic parameters, PDU offers concrete evidence that can substantiate or refute allegations in medicolegal cases and might mitigate subjective biases that might otherwise influence legal judgments. Also accurate differentiation between organic and psychogenic ED aids in presenting an informed medical perspective in legal contexts [12].

However, while PDU might be useful in medicolegal cases, ethical considerations are paramount. Clinicians must ensure patient consent, privacy, and the responsible use of PDU data within the legal framework. Ethical practices safeguard both the patient's well-being and the integrity of the legal process.

6.4 Prognosis

The integration of PDU into the diagnostic and therapeutic approach of ED provides valuable prognostic insights for both patients and healthcare professionals. In fact, PDU contributes to the prediction of treatment response by evaluating penile vascularization. It is also possible to suggest that serial assessments of penile blood flow using PDU enable healthcare professionals to gauge the progression of arterial insufficiency over time. This longitudinal data aids in tailoring treatment plans, optimizing medical management, and eventually enhancing patient satisfaction. This latter aspect is of utmost importance. PDU aids in predicting the likelihood of treatment success and improved erectile function, ultimately influencing patient satisfaction. By offering insights into the expected outcomes of various interventions, PDU empowers patients to make informed decisions about their treatment options [13].

On the other hand, the actual value of PDU in adding prognostic value to patients with ED has been questioned [14, 15]. As satisfactory response to PDE5-I theoretically confirms the presence of adequate arterial inflow and veno-occlusive mechanisms, these authors debate the actual need for PDU confirmation [15]. Also, in these studies the authors use the absence of significant correlation between any given PDU parameter and long-term IIEF scores. The problem in that approach is that it is impossible to account for the nuances in the PDU procedure, and analyzing the parameters alone diminishes the potential value of this diagnostic modality in patient management. Moreover, throughout this chapter, PDU applicability has been extensively discussed, suggesting that in many ways PDU may be valuable in different scenarios.

6.5 Translation from PDE5i to More Invasive Therapies

In cases where PDE5i therapy fails to yield satisfactory results, PDU assists in identifying real non-responders to pharmacotherapy. In fact, a more profound understanding of the vascular component of ED may help in determining whether further investment in PDE5i salvage therapy is advisable.

Moreover, transitioning from PDE5i to more invasive therapeutic options is a critical juncture in the management of ED, and the objective data obtained during PDU examinations help clinicians recognize when a transition to more invasive therapies might be warranted.

By assessing penile blood flow responses to ICI, PDU offers insights into the likelihood of achieving satisfactory erectile function through this treatment modality. In fact, most patients tend to be more receptive to a diagnostic examination than to a long-term injectable therapy, which makes PDU examinations a resistance breaker. After performing PDU, many individuals become more receptive to the idea of penile injection therapy.

Finally, PDU can help identify patients who may benefit from penile prosthetic surgery. Before considering penile prosthesis implantation for the treatment of refractory ED, high-quality PDU with redosing strategies might be offered to ensure end-stage ED. In these cases, PDU might eventually serve as medical written documentation and an appealing argument to warrant medical insurance coverage for penile implant surgery.

6.6   Conclusions

PDU emerges as an invaluable asset in the comprehensive diagnosis and management of ED. This chapter has explored the multifaceted role of PDU in assessing vascular dynamics and therapeutic outcomes pertaining to ED.

As a noninvasive and dynamic imaging technique, PDU offers a range of benefits that contribute to enhanced patient care and improved treatment strategies. Although the generalized use of PDU is not recommended, it has been proven useful in special populations such as in younger patients or in patients with Peyronie's disease. Whether transitioning from phosphodiesterase type 5 inhibitors (PDE5i) to more invasive therapies or evaluating treatment response over time, PDU ensures that interventions are aligned with the individual's physiological profile.

As a prognostic tool, PDU aids in predicting treatment outcomes, long-term erectile function, and patient satisfaction. By offering insights into the success of interventions, PDU empowers both clinicians and patients to make informed decisions, optimizing therapeutic strategies and improving overall well-being.

As PDU enthusiasts, the authors believe that it elevates the field of sexual medicine as it provides accurate, objective, and dynamic data that guide diagnostics, treatment decisions, and prognostication of ED. Its role extends beyond diagnosis into personalized therapeutic strategies, enhancing patient care and contributing to improved quality of life for individuals struggling with ED.

References

1. Lue TF. Erectile dysfunction. N Engl J Med. 2000;342(24):1802–13.
2. Wilson SK, Cleves MA, Delk JR 2nd. Long-term followup of treatment for Peyronie's disease: modeling the penis over an inflatable penile prosthesis. J Urol. 2001;165(3):825–9.
3. Terris MK, Klaassen Z. Office-based ultrasound for the urologist. Urol Clin N Am. 2013;40(4):637–47.
4. Masterson TA 3rd, Efimenko IV, Nackeeran S, Parmar M, Ramasamy R. Discordant erectile function assessment between validated questionnaire scores and penile Doppler ultrasound in Peyronie's disease. Int J Impot Res. 2022;34(5):452–5.
5. Nashed A, Lokeshwar SD, Frech F, Mann U, Patel P. The efficacy of penile duplex ultrasound in erectile dysfunction management decision-making: a systematic review. Sex Med Rev. 2021;9(3):472–7.

6. Nehra A, Alterowitz R, Culkin DJ, Faraday MM, Hakim LS, Heidelbaugh JJ, et al. Peyronie's disease: AUA guideline. J Urol. 2015;194(3):745–53.
7. Carneiro F, Saito OC, Miranda EP. Standardization of penile hemodynamic evaluation through color duplex-Doppler ultrasound. Rev Assoc Med Bras (1992). 2020;66(9):1180–6.
8. Meller SM, Stilp E, Walker CN, Mena-Hurtado C. The link between vasculogenic erectile dysfunction, coronary artery disease, and peripheral artery disease: role of metabolic factors and endovascular therapy. J Invasive Cardiol. 2013;25(6):313–9.
9. Yannas D, Frizza F, Vignozzi L, Corona G, Maggi M, Rastrelli G. Erectile dysfunction is a hallmark of cardiovascular disease: unavoidable matter of fact or opportunity to improve men's health? J Clin Med. 2021;10(10):2221.
10. Gupta N, Herati A, Gilbert BR. Penile Doppler ultrasound predicting cardiovascular disease in men with erectile dysfunction. Curr Urol Rep. 2015;16(3):16.
11. Hekal IA, Mosbah A, El-Bahnasawy MS, El-Assmy A, Shaaban A. Penile haemodynamic changes in post-radical cystectomy patients. Int J Androl. 2011;34(1):27–32.
12. Ozkara H, Aşicioglu F, Alici B, Akkuş E, Hattat H. Retrospective analysis of medicolegal cases and evaluation for erectile function. Am J Forensic Med Pathol. 1999;20(2):145–9.
13. Patel P, Masterson T, Ramasamy R. Penile duplex: clinical indications and application. Int J Impot Res. 2019;31(4):298–9.
14. Morgado A, Dinis P, Silva CM. Is there a role for bilateral peak systolic velocity readings in a penile duplex ultrasound? Andrologia. 2019;51(8):e13297.
15. Morgado A, Diniz P, Silva CM. Is there a point to performing a penile duplex ultrasound? J Sex Med. 2019;16(10):1574–80.

Chapter 7
Pharmacotherapy for Inducing an Erection

7.1   Introduction

Inducing an erection is perhaps the most significant challenge during penile hemo-dynamic studies. After the learning curve for the adjustment of parameters in the ultrasound device, the technical aspects of scanning the arteries are usually a straightforward procedure. On the other hand, each patient will display a particular clinical feature of erectile dysfunction (ED) and will require an individualized approach to obtaining a rigid erection. Moreover, complications during penile Doppler ultrasound are always related to the erection-induction process, which requires extreme caution throughout the examination. Therefore, an adequate man-agement of intracavernous therapy of vasoactive agents is a requirement for high-quality examinations.

Although intracavernous pharmacotherapy (ICT) can be directly offered an ED treatment option with progressive dose titration, we believe the performing penile Doppler ultrasound (PDU) is the best option to transition the patients from oral to injectable. Most patients will demonstrate less resistance to perform PDU than to start long-term ICT right away.

7.2   Historical Background

Since the historical introduction of papaverine in the early 1980s, ICT has emerged as the first effective medication-based treatment for ED. At that time, the intracav-ernous route was considered a minimally invasive approach and revolutionized medical treatment to manage ED. Also, the application of ICT to induce an erection for diagnostic purposes during penile hemodynamic studies has been first described

E. d. P. Miranda, F. Carneiro, *Penile Color Duplex-Doppler Ultrasound in
Erectile Dysfunction Diagnosis and Management*,
https://doi.org/10.1007/978-3-031-55649-4_7

in 1985. In the mid-1990s, alprostadil for ICT became the first drug approved for ED, while combined pharmacotherapy has been available in the market since the mid-1980s [1].

ICT remained very popular up until late 1990s with the introduction of phosphodiesterase type 5 inhibitors (PDE5i) to the market. However, clinical data gathered to date suggest that ICT remains a viable and effective therapy, particularly for individuals who are poor responders to PDE5 inhibitors, those with contraindications, or those who cannot tolerate them [2, 3].

7.3 Vasoactive Agents

For an erection to occur, sexual arousal usually triggers the production and release of nitric oxide (NO) from nerve endings and vascular endothelial cells located in the penis, which is facilitated by nitric oxide synthase (NOS). Once produced, NO quickly diffuses into the corpora cavernosa and activates guanylyl cyclase (GC), an enzyme that converts guanosine-50-triphosphate to cyclic guanosine monophosphate (cGMP). As a result, cGMP levels increase, which stimulates cGMP-dependent protein kinase, leading to a decrease in intracellular calcium. Ultimately, smooth muscle relaxation occurs, resulting in blood accumulation into the penis by increased arterial inflow and decreased venous outflow. The process is terminated by the breakdown of cGMP by PDE5. PDE5is work by hindering the degradation of cGMP, thereby keeping cGMP levels elevated, and facilitating a penile erection (Fig. 7.1).

However, it is important to note that PDE5is are not erectogenic drugs and require the presence of sexual arousal and an intact nerve function to allow NO production [4].

ICT refers to the administration of vasoactive substances through injection into the corpora cavernosa using a fine needle. The most common substances used in ICT nowadays include prostaglandin E1, papaverine, phentolamine, and occasionally atropine. These substances can act alone or in conjunction to facilitate the attainment of an erection even in the absence of sexual stimuli and independently from the NO/cGMP pathway [4].

7.3.1 Prostaglandin E1

Prostaglandin E1 (PGE1) also known as alprostadil causes potent relaxation of the human corpora cavernosa through stimulation of receptors and targets membrane-bound adenylyl cyclase (AC) to increase cAMP. In the cellular cascade, the cAMP pathway activates protein kinase A and similarly to cGMP will promote smooth muscle relaxation.

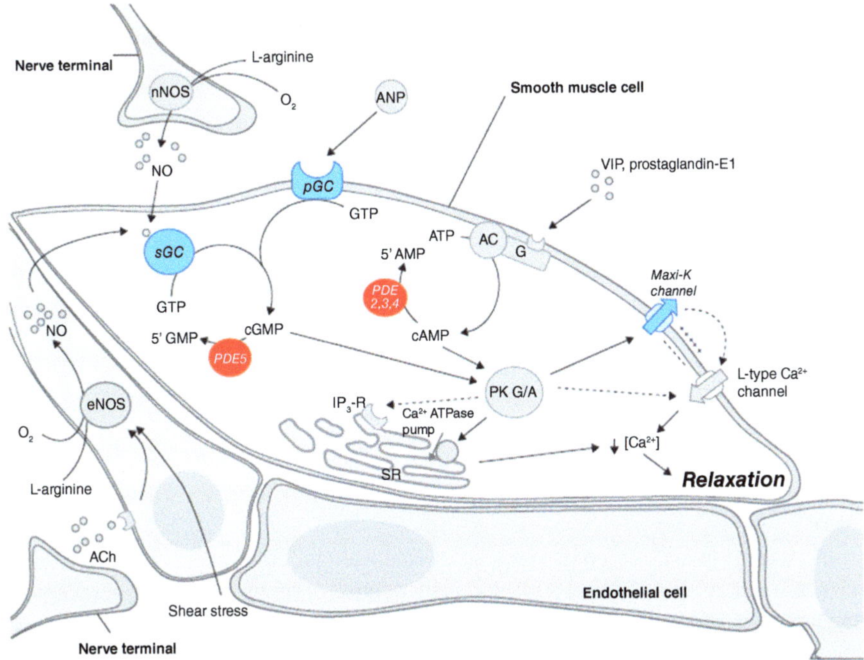

Fig. 7.1 Pathways of smooth muscle relaxation. (Adapted from Albersen et al.)

PGE1 doses usually vary between 2.5–40 mcg and will provide an optimal erectile response conducive for sexual satisfaction in more than 70% and a significant increase in rigidity scores in 90% of men with ED of psychogenic, organic, or mixed etiology [1]. Over the past decades, extensive clinical data has supported the safety and efficacy of PGE1 as a vasoactive agent for ED monotherapy. The dose of PGE1 can be eventually increased up to 60 mg safely, and it is generally well tolerated, with only a few side effects.

A mild form of local pain has been reported in 11% after injection of PGE1. It is most commonly seen in patients with neurogenic ED, most notably in post radical prostatectomy or diabetic patients and might indicate some degree of nerve damage. Although this diffuse pain might decrease over time, it is usually recommended that PGE1 be avoided in these situations.

7.3.2 Papaverine

Papaverine was the first agent discovered to improve penile erections in ICT and is obtained from the opium poppy (*Papaver somniferum*). It is a nonspecific phosphodiesterase inhibitor that increases intracellular cAMP along with cGMP levels and inhibits voltage-dependent calcium channels promoting relaxation of smooth muscle in the sinusoids and dilatation of helicine arterioles.

The risk of general systemic effects is low in most cases because the locally injected papaverine is minimally transmitted through the corporeal venous system. However, some rare cases of elevated hepatic enzymes and hepatotoxicity have been reported. The drug is considered cost-effective within the pharmacologic dose range of 10–60 mg. Conversely, the primary drawbacks associated with this agent are usually associated with higher risks of developing corporeal fibrosis. This side effect is believed to result from the low acidity (pH 3–4) of papaverine. Currently, papaverine is primarily reserved for use in combination with other vasoactive drugs, allowing for lower concentrations and an advantageous diagnostic and therapeutic synergy in terms of safety and efficacy [5].

7.3.3 Phentolamine

In the flaccid penis, the contraction of cavernosal smooth muscles is attributed to α1-adrenoreceptor activity. Phentolamine injection inhibits these adrenoreceptors and activates NO synthase, leading to an induced erection. However, due to its nonselective α-adrenoreceptor inhibition, phentolamine may cause several adverse events, including reflex tachycardia and hypotension. As phentolamine does not provide a significant therapeutic outcome as monotherapy, it is recommended primarily for combination therapies.

7.3.4 Combination Therapy

Several combinations of intracavernous vasoactive agents have been introduced. The rationale behind the use of combination therapies is to enable supply of the erectile process by different pathways in a synergic fashion. Table 7.1 displays the most common intracavernous agents and its pharmacologic effects.

Various combinations are currently available including those with 2 (Bimix), 3 (Trimix), or 4 agents (Quadrimix). Note that combinations are possible with

Table 7.1 List of the most common vasoactive agents and their mechanism of action

Vasoactive agent	Mechanisms of action
Papaverine	Nonspecific phosphodiesterase inhibitor inhibits voltage-dependent calcium channels
Phentolamine	Inhibits α1-adrenoreceptor activity of contractile response of the cavernosum
Prostaglandin E1	Stimulates membrane-bound adenylyl cyclase to increase cAMP
Atropine	Blocks the anti-erectile arm of the cholinergic pathway in the human cavernosum

different agents and dosages, especially in Bimix formulas, which can be compounded with or without PGE1. In theory, more components and a higher concentration per mL of each drug will contribute to a higher potency of ICT. Therefore, there are multiple available combinations that may vary according to country and/or region, manufacturer, and physician preference.

As an example of a successful three-drug approach, PGE1 activates the cAMP pathway, while papaverine blocks phosphodiesterases, thus prolonging the functional efficacy of both cAMP and cGMP, and phentolamine counteracts the adrenoreceptor-mediated contractile response of the cavernosum, completing a more potent induction of smooth muscle relaxation.

7.3.4.1 Bimix

A combination of papaverine with the competitive a-adrenoreceptor blocker, phentolamine, is the most popular bimix preparation. The addition of phentolamine decreases arterial resistance and promotes vasodilatation in synergy with papaverine. As mentioned early, a bimix combination of PGE1 and phentolamine is also effective and is preferred for those who want to avoid the use of papaverine because of its pharmacological properties.

The addition of PGE1 to the combination will create issues regarding storage of the vials. Ideally, vials containing PGE1 should be refrigerated at temperatures around 2–8 °C, since it is the least stable of the drug components at room temperature. It has been suggested that 8% of PGE1 loss occurred in 5 days at room temperature [6].

7.3.4.2 Trimix

Trimix combinations have been shown to increase efficacy in penile hemodynamic studies because it is effective and more suitable in poor responders to PGE1 monotherapy. Although many formulations of trimix are available, perhaps a mixture consisting of papaverine 30 mg/mL, phentolamine 1 mg/mL, and PGE1 10 mcg/mL is most commonly reported in the literature. Due to stability concerns associated with the combination of agents, there are no commercially available preparations for trimix. Compounding pharmacies must reconstitute the mixture and provide storage instructions to ensure its shelf-life protection.

For long-term ICT, trimix appears to perform better in subjective preference in the context of rigidity enhancement and sexual satisfaction, being twice as effective as PGE1 (40 mcg) monotherapy with minimal pain [7]. As mentioned earlier, it seems that the combination effectively targeted the different pathways involved in the erectile mechanism. A study evaluating 122 men using ICT for at least 6 months has demonstrated that during a long-term follow-up period of 25 months, it was found that 65% of individuals who did not respond well to PDE5 inhibitors were able to successfully continue with ICT, of whom 85% were trimix users [8].

7.3.4.3 Quadrimix

This preparation exemplifies a multidrug combination therapy aiming superior efficacy for more severe cases of ED. It is very unlikely that such a combination is required for standard PDU examinations.

The idea is to add atropine to the trimix mixture in order to increase pharmacological potency. However, the usefulness of atropine, a known anticholinergic agent, has been subject to questioning, as acetylcholine has relaxation properties in the smooth muscle. The rationale is that atropine may block the anti-erectile arm of the cholinergic pathway in the human corpora cavernosa, thereby facilitating the non-adrenergic non-cholinergic and endothelium-derived relaxing factor mechanisms involved in the erectile process [9].

Quadrimix had an enhanced therapeutic potential and safety margin, typical of a multidrug synergism. However, its clinical applicability is usually reserved for restoration of satisfactory erectile capacity in patients with more severe ED and some degree of veno-occlusive dysfunction demonstrated in penile Doppler studies [10].

7.3.4.4 High Concentration Preparations

The actual dose delivered to the penis takes into account two variables: the concentration and the volume of the drugs within each formulation. So, in order to optimize clinical response with any given ICT, one should either increase the applied volume or chose a higher potency combination. Initially increasing the volume is the most logical solution that will most likely provide a beneficial effect. However, upgrading the potency of the drug might be more cost effective for patients requiring very high volumes in each injection. Especially because volumes >0.5 mL might lead to more long-term complications such as extravasation of the fluid that might lead to palpable nodules, among others.

Therefore, it is possible to maximize the concentration in each preparation, which is commonly referred to using the prefix "super" (superbimix, supertrimix, etc.). These preparations usually accommodate up to 2–3 times higher concentrations per milliliter, sometimes respecting the maximal solubility of each individual component to avoid eventual precipitation. Although a systemic effect of hypotension is possible in higher concentration of ICT, it is not commonly seen in clinical practice [11].

7.4 How to Choose the Ideal Agent?

In fact, there is no such a thing as an ideal agent. For the purpose of performing PDU studies, the examiner must choose an agent or combination that allows complete smooth muscle relaxation, which is usually obtained with redosing protocols. A practical list of recommended preparations is described in Table 7.2. Increasing the volume by multiple dosing might compensate for lower concentrations in the combination of vasoactive agents. On the other hand, one of the main limitations of

Table 7.2 List of the most common combination therapies for performing intracavernous therapy and penile Doppler ultrasound studies with suggested dosage

Combination therapy	Dose and components
Trimix	Papaverine 30 mg/mL, phentolamine 1 mg/mL, and alprostadil 10 mcg/mL
Bimix	Papaverine 30 mg/mL, phentolamine 1 mg/mL
Supertrimix[a]	Papaverine 50 mg/mL, phentolamine 5 mg/mL, and alprostadil 20 mcg/mL
(Super)Quadrimix[a]	Papaverine 20 mg/mL, phentolamine 3 mg/mL, and alprostadil 40 mcg/mL, atropine 0.1 mg/mL

[a]*These combinations might vary dramatically in different markets and compound pharmacies*

the literature regarding PDU examinations is the lack of standardized protocols. Therefore, we advocate the routine use of trimix for all penile hemodynamic studies, because it gathers most favorable characteristics of potency and safety at the same time that allows extensive redosing protocols. More specifically, we suggest the combination of papaverine 30 mg/mL, phentolamine 1 mg/mL, and PGE1 10 mg/mL, which is the most commonly reported in the literature and the most commonly found globally [12].

Although the use of PGE1 monotherapy is also a possibility because it has less risk of prolonged erection/priapism, we believe that it should not be the first choice. Not only because it is less efficient, especially in more severe cases of ED, but also because a considerable redosing strategy is more troublesome and might be even painful as a result of very high concentration of prostaglandin. A poor response to PGE1 testing has been observed in men with diabetes, metabolic syndrome, and low testosterone levels, which is a population of men that would most likely benefit from PDU examination. The use of supertrimix or quadrimix is also not necessary if one is considering scaling up to 1 mL of the traditional trimix.

For the purpose of long-term ICT, the rationale is somehow different. We usually recommend PDU examination prior initiation of ICT, though we acknowledge that it is not a requirement in all cases. In such cases, all the patients will have a first experience with trimix in a standardized concentration. According to the erectile response, patients will be titrated to higher or lower potency preparations, with aims to maintain the minimal volume necessary for a satisfactory erectile function. For those requiring very high volumes (>0.5 mL) of trimix, supertrimix or quadrimix is offered. If penile pain or tenderness is reported at the time of PDU, or if the patient had prolonged erections that required reversal with very low volumes of trimix, then bimix preparations without PGE1 would be more suitable in such cases.

7.5   Redosing Protocol

As mentioned earlier in this chapter, each patient has a particular set of characteristic that will need an individualized approach to obtaining a rigid erection. In other words, if a standard dose were given to all patients undergoing PDU examination, a significant number of individuals would not achieve complete smooth muscle relaxation, which could be inferred by their best quality erection (BQE) possible. The BQE refers to the highest grade of erection that the patient has experienced in any scenario at home, whether masturbatory, sexual, or even a nocturnal erection. These scenarios typically involve less anxiety than the PDU settings. If the patient is unable to achieve a BQE, it is advisable to administer additional vasoactive medication, unless hemodynamics are already normal [12]. Therefore, it is very important to establish a progressive redosing protocol that allows every patient a chance of having their BQE without overdosing and increasing the risk of priapism.

The first step is to select 1 or 2 combinations of vasoactive agents to be used routinely in order to facilitate experience-acquiring process. We recommend using trimix (papaverine 30 mg/mL, phentolamine 1 mg/mL, and alprostadil 10 mcg/mL) for the vast majority of patients, unless the patients have known pain elicited by alprostadil or are known users of a more potent combination of ICT. In the latter, we recommend using bimix (papaverine 30 mg/mL, phentolamine 1 mg/mL), and in the former, perhaps the best idea is to use the patients' regular ICT combination. A step-by-step guide is described in Table 7.3.

Although there is no maximal dose of trimix or bimix allowed, we have set the limit of 1 mL of each medication, which should be ideally delivered in up to 3 injections in 10-min intervals. This decision is based on the fact that usually 1 mL syringes are used for long-term ICT, which makes it at least viable to prescribe the same dose utilized in the PDU examination. Injecting more than 3 times in 10-min intervals would make the examination excessively time consuming.

The initial dose should be 0.05–0.1 mL (5–10 units) of trimix depending on the patient age, risk factors, and/or severity of ED. This relatively low initial dose is important to avoid giving higher dose for patients with extreme sensitivity to the ICT combination. From this point on, the redosing strategy could follow (1) a predetermined sequence or (2) could vary according to patient rigidity.

The first option could be considered a more conservative approach. For example, the examiner is willing to deliver up to 3 fixed doses of 0.1, 0.2, and 0.2 mL of trimix beforehand. In this case, a total of 0.5 mL of trimix would be given, which is considered a relatively high dose, but would not reach the maximum dosing of 1 mL. This is a good strategy for providers who are not very familiar with redosing strategies and rigidity evaluation. On the second approach, there are no previous

Table 7.3 Step by step recommendation of a highly effective redosing protocol

Protocol
1. Provide a relaxant and cozy environment to decrease patients' adrenalin levels
2. Inject 0.05–0.1 mL (5–10 units) of trimix (papaverine 30 mg/mL, phentolamine 1 mg/mL, and alprostadil 10 mcg/mL) or bimix (papaverine 30 mg/mL, phentolamine 1 mg/mL) according to patient characteristics
3. Perform erection rigidity assessment in 10-min intervals to evaluate the need for redosing in up to 3 injections and a maximal dose of 1 mL
4. Redosing should be ceased if the patient has achieved a rigid erection (Erection Hardness Score—EHS 4/4 or 8/10). If not possible, at least his best quality erection (BQE) is desirable

limits, and the decision is made as the examination is performed. For example, the examiner could start at 0.1 mL, and after 10 min, the patient is displaying an erection 1/10. As a result, he decides to give a second injection of 0.3 mL and the result was 4/10. Then he decides to give a third injection of 0.6 mL and final erection 6/10, really close to his BQE. If this exact patient were given 0.5 mL only according to the fixed-dose strategy, he would probably have to repeat his examination or be tried with higher doses of ICT in the clinical follow-up. On the other hand, the scalable dosing up to 1 mL could lead to overdosing requiring intensive reversal strategies, in case of failure to perform a correct evaluation of rigidity.

Redosing medication is usually not required when the patient has obtained a rigid erection (Erection HardnessScore—EHS 4/4 or 8/10), his BQE, or if the maximum dose of 1 mL has been administered.

7.6 Application Technique

A correct application technique is a requirement for the correct conduction of PDU studies, as demonstrated in Fig. 7.2. Although relatively simple for most urologists, some radiologists might encounter some difficulties. Special attention is required in patients with severe obesity, buried penis, or other anatomic abnormalities of the penis. First it is important to perform palpation of the penis under stretch, to identify plaques that might prevent correct entrance of the needle. The penis should be kept under stretch to confer stability to the injection site. The needle should be pushed until it has certainly entered the corpora cavernosa, and the medication should be applied without resistance. After the injection, apply gentle pressure at the site of injection to avoid hematoma formation and fluid extravasation as much as possible, ideally around 10 s. For patients under antiplatelet or anticoagulant therapy, longer periods of 30 s are recommended. In cases where injection difficulties may be foreseen, we recommend injecting 0.01–0.02 mL of air along with the medication to generate hyperechoic images within the corpora cavernosa that can be seen using the ultrasound probe during initial scanning of the penis to confirm that the medication was delivered in the right place.

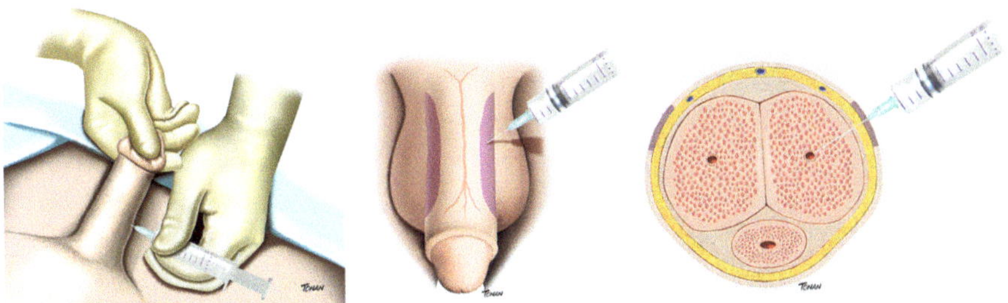

Fig. 7.2 Demonstration of correct penile injection technique with correct grasp of the penis, ideal injection site, and syringe angle

When long-term ICT is recommended, patients will need to be trained for self-administration of penile injection therapy. During training sessions, instructions must stress the significance of maintaining aseptic measures and correct utilization of an ultrathin needle for administering the medication into the corpora cavernosa through the lateral aspect (3 or 9 o'clock) avoiding the perforation of superficial veins. Caution is also required to prevent accidental harm to the mid-dorsal structures. For patients who are nervous about administering manual needle injections, automatic self-injection devices can be beneficial. In individuals with poor manual dexterity, morbid obesity, or impaired visual acuity, self-administration of vasoactive agents can be challenging, and sometimes the sexual partner has to be trained to perform the injections or the patient may not be a candidate for ICT at all. Training sessions can enhance adherence to the self-injection regimen and minimize the risk of complications. The physician has the responsibility of determining a suitable dose of the vasoactive agent during an office visit, along with providing explicit instructions on the frequency of self-administration for use at home. It usually takes some time for the patients to become proficient in self-injection of ICT programs because there are many different possibilities for errors, as suggested in Fig. 7.3. Therefore, a close follow-up during the first steps and an open communication line are warranted in order to avoid complications and ensure adequate adhesion rates.

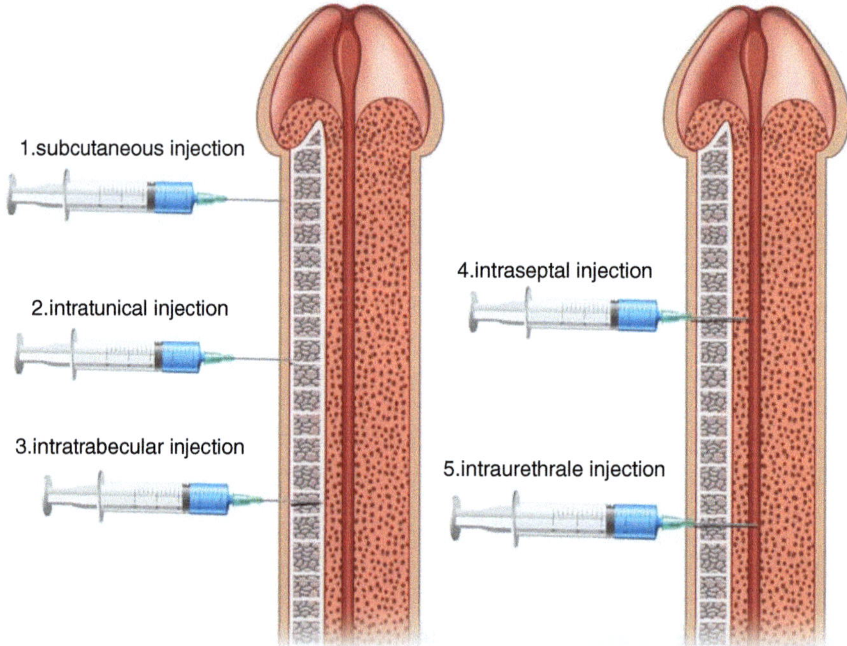

Fig. 7.3 Potential errors during intracavernous injections. (Adapted from [11])

7.7 Principles of Long-Term Intracavernosal Therapy

Men who have contraindications to the use of PDE5i, prefer not to take an oral medication, or find that PDE5i is inadequate or ineffective may choose the ICT approach to treat ED. Similarly, during early rehabilitation after prostatectomy, vasoactive drugs are beneficial in facilitating the recovery of spontaneous erections [13]. These patients should be informed regarding benefits and risks/burdens of this treatment strategy. Also, it is very important that patients take co-responsibility to follow specific medical orders, because many of the complications are consequence of inability to follow pre-established protocols.

Men considering ICT should first have an in-office injection test to start titration protocols [2], which we believe should be an ideal session for PDU examination. Once the initial dose has been defined, titration should be adjusted according to the rigidity and duration of the erection. The goal is to obtain an erection rigid enough for penetration (>Erection Hardness Score grade 3—EHS 3 or >60% erection) for about 1 h. Dose increases should be done gradually with dose variation of about 20–50% according to clinical response. If erection duration is over 1.5 h, there should be considerations about decreasing the dose.

A specific priapism plan should be agreed with the patient in case of erections lasting >3 h, so detumescence maneuvers should be started with no delays after 4 h of duration.

Patients could eventually be safely trained for self-injection of sympathomimetics for erection reversal in selected cases [14].

7.8 Contraindications and Complications

Although there is a classic list of absolute contraindication for the use of ICT, to date it is possible to assume these have become relative. In other words, there is no formal contraindication for performing PDU evaluation or to initiate cautious ICT for patients with ED. However, an extra caution is required in men who are at risk to develop spontaneous priapism, such as those with hematological disorders such as polycythemia, leukemia, multiple myeloma, and sickle cell disease. Bleeding disorders or use anticoagulant therapy does not necessarily rule out the possibility of ICT. In such cases, patients should be counseled to apply longer pressure after each injection and should be advised about the increased risk of bruising and hematomas [15].

There are known complications associated to PDU and/or ICT, which include possible infections on the injection site, ecchymosis, or hematoma formation due to its invasive route of administration. Penile bleeding and ecchymoses have been reported in up to 8%, and systemic side effects like including dizziness and syncope are very rarely reported. Pain is a prevalent side effect of ICT. However, it is important to differentiate regular pain following a needle prick on the penis to that related to pharmacological effects of prostaglandin. The former is resolved with time and improvement of the application technique, while the latter require change in the medication or combination of choice.

The most feared complications are priapism and cavernosal fibrosis, which are also considered infrequent with overall prevalence <10% [1]. These are much more related to the long-term use of ICT and not directly to PDU. Although there are many studies suggesting that these rates are usually associated to the agent or combination that is used, we believe that these complications are more related to the mode of use and the quality of care the patient receives than to the pharmacological effect of the medication itself.

7.8.1   Priapism

As the potency and dosage of vasoactive agents increase, there is a greater likelihood of experiencing pharmacologically induced prolonged erection and priapism. Although reports have demonstrated the lowest priapism rates with PGE1 of about 1.8% [11], there are ICT programs with trimix with priapism rates <1%. If penile rigidity persists for longer than 4–6 h, medical intervention is necessary, which typically involves an intracavernous injection of a sympathomimetic drug (such as phenylephrine, etilefrine, or epinephrine) with or without needle aspiration of the trapped blood.

This is the most serious complication associated with ICT/PDU and is fortunately rather uncommon when strict quality criteria are followed. To mitigate the risk of priapism, it is crucial to identify the suitable medication dosage and provide instructions to the patient regarding dose titration.

7.8.2   Penile Fibrosis

Penile fibrosis defined as the development of plaque, nodules, or penile deformities has been reported with use of ICT with considerable range across medications (4.5–13%) [11]. However, although indirect signs of penile fibrosis have been classically found in men on long-term ICT, this causal association remains controversial [16].

Although in vitro studies have demonstrated a cytotoxic impact on cavernosal smooth muscle cells, endothelial cells, and fibroblasts, animal studies have revealed that any structural changes are typically limited to the injection site and do not have a significant effect on penile structure. Similarly, a causal association between ICT and Peyronie's disease (PD) has not been established. It remains unclear whether ICT therapy genuinely increases the risk of developing PD compared to the risk for an age-matched population not on ICT.

Retrospective uncontrolled studies have shown that fibrotic changes have a low incidence and are typically limited to the injection site, often going unnoticed by patients and resulting in no clinically significant curvature. In fact, a significant proportion of these fibrotic or nodular lesions have been documented to resolve spontaneously in two large, multicenter, long-term follow-up studies conducted worldwide [11].

Experience shows that most patients on ICT will develop no significant penile changes in terms of fibrosis. Eventually, those presenting for PDU are diagnosed with unnoticed PD because of lack of rigidity during erections. Fact is that patients requiring ICT may share common risk factor for the development of fibrosis, and this controversy might remain for undetermined periods of time. If a patient on ICT develops any signs of fibrotic changes, it is important to recognize potential modifiable risk factors such as injection technique and medication volume and eventually suggest change in medication combination profile or even avoid ICT momentarily to prevent progression.

7.9 Conclusions

ICT can be considered the cornerstone to assess penile hemodynamics during PDU in the evaluation of vascular causes for ED. Furthermore, they can be indicated for ED treatment in multiple scenarios regardless of etiology. Practitioners who perform PDU should be acquainted with the variety of vasoactive agents available both as monotherapy and in combination therapy, which are designed to accentuate different pathways contributing to the erectile process and optimally enhance arterial and smooth muscle relaxation. They should also be familiar with the most significant pitfalls and complications related to this pharmacotherapy. Complications regarding ICT for both therapeutic and diagnostic purposes are infrequent and preventable in most cases with proper medical counsel and follow-up.

References

1. Hatzimouratidis K, Salonia A, Adaikan G, Buvat J, Carrier S, El-Meliegy A, et al. Pharmacotherapy for erectile dysfunction: recommendations from the fourth international consultation for sexual medicine (ICSM 2015). J Sex Med. 2016;13(4):465–88.
2. Burnett AL, Nehra A, Breau RH, Culkin DJ, Faraday MM, Hakim LS, et al. Erectile dysfunction: AUA guideline. J Urol. 2018;200(3):633–41.
3. Salonia A, Bettocchi C, Boeri L, Capogrosso P, Carvalho J, Cilesiz NC, et al. European Association of Urology Guidelines on Sexual and Reproductive Health-2021 update: male sexual dysfunction. Eur Urol. 2021;80(3):333–57.
4. Yafi FA, Jenkins L, Albersen M, Corona G, Isidori AM, Goldfarb S, et al. Erectile dysfunction. Nat Rev Dis Prim. 2016;2:16003.

5. Kilic M, Serefoglu EC, Ozdemir AT, Balbay MD. The actual incidence of papaverine-induced priapism in patients with erectile dysfunction following penile colour Doppler ultrasonography. Andrologia. 2010;42(1):1–4.
6. Trissel LA, Zhang Y. Long-term stability of trimix: a three-drug injection used to treat erectile dysfunction. Int J Pharm Compd. 2004;8(3):231–5.
7. Bechara A, Casabé A, Chéliz G, Romano S, Fredotovich N. Prostaglandin E1 versus mixture of prostaglandin E1, papaverine and phentolamine in nonresponders to high papaverine plus phentolamine doses. J Urol. 1996;155(3):913–4.
8. Hsiao W, Bennett N, Guhring P, Narus J, Mulhall JP. Satisfaction profiles in men using intra-cavernosal injection therapy. J Sex Med. 2011;8(2):512–7.
9. Adaikan PG, Karim SM, Kottegoda SR, Ratnam SS. Cholinoreceptors in the corpus cavernosum muscle of the human penis. J Auton Pharmacol. 1983;3(2):107–11.
10. Fayez AH, El-Khayat Y, Hosny H, Zaki S, Shamloul R. A study of the possible effects of repeated intracorporeal self-injection of vasoactive drugs in patients with elevated end diastolic velocity during pharmacopenile duplex ultrasonography. Cent Eur J Urol. 2013;66(2):210–4.
11. Porst H, Burnett A, Brock G, Ghanem H, Giuliano F, Glina S, et al. SOP conservative (medical and mechanical) treatment of erectile dysfunction. J Sex Med. 2013;10(1):130–71.
12. Nascimento B, Miranda EP, Terrier JE, Carneiro F, Mulhall JP. A critical analysis of methodology pitfalls in Duplex Doppler ultrasound in the evaluation of patients with erectile dysfunction: technical and interpretation deficiencies. J Sex Med. 2020;17(8):1416–22.
13. Polito M, d'Anzeo G, Conti A, Muzzonigro G. Erectile rehabilitation with intracavernous alprostadil after radical prostatectomy: refusal and dropout rates. BJU Int. 2012;110(11 Pt C):E954–7.
14. Teloken C, Ribeiro EP, Chammas M Jr, Teloken PE, Souto CA. Intracavernosal etilefrine self-injection therapy for recurrent priapism: one decade of follow-up. Urology. 2005;65(5):1002.
15. Belew D, Klaassen Z, Lewis RW. Intracavernosal injection for the diagnosis, evaluation, and treatment of erectile dysfunction: a review. Sex Med Rev. 2015;3(1):11–23.
16. Tal R, Mulhall JP. Intracavernosal injections and fibrosis: myth or reality? BJU Int. 2008;102(5):525–6.

Chapter 8
Penile Rigidity Assessment

8.1 Introduction

Penile rigidity assessment is an important step during hemodynamic studies. Eventually, a subjective assessment of erectile function might function for the purpose of managing erectile dysfunction (ED) in clinical practice. However, during penile Doppler ultrasound (PDU) examination, a more objective, reliable, and reproducible analysis of the penile erection is warranted. The clinical decision for redosing of intracavernous vasoactive agents during PDU depends on a reliable way to assess rigidity and inquiring about the patient's best quality erection (BQE). Moreover, it is important to remind the reader that the quantification of penile hardness is also critical in various clinical scenarios, such as comparing various surgical options for Peyronie's disease, evaluating the efficacy of recently developed therapies for ED, and providing guidance to patients prior to procedure that might lead to cavernous nerves damage [1]. The goal of this chapter is to provide a comprehensive overview of the available tools for the assessment of penile rigidity and provide practical recommendations for their clinical use.

8.2 Erection Biomechanics

The penis might be considered a column formed by three solid circular cylinders: two cavernous bodies and one spongiosal body. The mechanism of erection physiology leads to an increase of intracavernosal pressure when the veno-occlusive mechanism is functioning. This pressure creates radial rigidity of the penis, allowing it to resist deformation when subjected to circumferential pressure.

© The Author(s), under exclusive license to Springer Nature
Switzerland AG 2024
E. d. P. Miranda, F. Carneiro, *Penile Color Duplex-Doppler Ultrasound in
Erectile Dysfunction Diagnosis and Management*,
https://doi.org/10.1007/978-3-031-55649-4_8

On the other hand, axial rigidity is a more complex concept and is considered a critical biomechanical property of the penis. It is defined as the ability to overcome the axial compression forces that when applied to the glans of the erect penis results in a pronounced curve that would result in buckling of the erect shaft. In other words, axial rigidity allows the penis to withstand compressive loads, such as those experienced during intromission and pelvic thrusting [1]. Axial rigidity of the penis is determined by radial rigidity, mechanical properties of the erectile tissue, and penile geometry [2].

In summary, from a mechanical engineering point of view, the hardness of an erection is an indication of the axial rigidity of the penis. Successful vaginal or anal intromission depends on the penile ability to maintain adequate axial rigidity to sustain collapsing or buckling forces [3, 4]. During PDU examinations, it is important to be aware of these distinct concepts for an adequate assessment of penile rigidity.

8.3 Measures of Erectile Function

During the evolution of sexual medicine, many tools have been developed to provide a comprehensive assessment of erectile function. These tools include validated questionnaires, intracavernosal injection testing, PDU itself, nocturnal penile tumescence testing, axial rigidity assessment with digital inflection rigidometer, shear wave elastography, and virtual touch, among others [1]. However, it is important to mention that these instruments will evaluate different aspects of penile erections. During penile hemodynamic studies, it is important to use instruments that evaluate both radial and axial rigidity. Therefore, it is possible to infer that nocturnal penile tumescence testing, which measures overnight radial rigidity alone, is not helpful for performing PDU. The International Index for Erectile Function (IIEF) itself, which may be eventually useful in the clinical assessment of ED and might aid in the indication of PDU, is also not relevant in the PDU technique. A more detailed discussion of these nuances is provided in the following items of this section.

8.3.1 Validated Questionnaires

The least invasive method for practitioners to obtain information about erectile hardness is through validated questionnaires, which have proven to be useful in quantifying the patient's assessment of their erection and providing insights into treatment strategies. Several questionnaires are available, but the International Index of Erectile Function (IIEF) has been validated across diverse ethnic and geographic contexts and has shown strong internal consistency, test–retest reproducibility,

Table 8.1 ED classification according to IIEF Erectile Function Domain

IIEF category	Scores
Severe	6–10
Moderate	11–16
Mild to moderate	17–21
Mild	22–25
No erectile dysfunction	26–30

**Minimum score for patient with sexual activity 6. Patients without attempts of sexual activity scores 0 in each question, with a total score of 0*

sensitivity, and specificity in multiple studies, being the most widely used in the clinical and research settings.

The IIEF is a patient-reported outcome measure that assesses multiple domains of male sexual function, including erectile function, orgasm, libido or desire, sexual satisfaction, and overall satisfaction. It contains the IIEF Erectile Function Domain (EFD) or IIEF-6, which is the primary diagnostic tool to evaluate changes in ED severity over the last 4 weeks of sexual activity. The IIEF-EFD contains six questions covering frequency of erection, firmness of erection, maintenance frequency, ability to achieve penetration, maintenance ability, and erection confidence. Respondents score each question from 1 (very low) to 5 (very high) based on the prior 4 weeks. The final score ranges and classification of ED are demonstrated in Table 8.1.

There is an abridged IIEF alternative, the Sexual Health Inventory for Men (SHIM) or IIEF-5. Although it is widely used and has good validity, it combines four questions of rigidity evaluation with a sexual satisfaction question within the last 6 months of sexual activity [5]. So, for the purpose evaluating penile rigidity in the clinical scenario, the authors suggest that the IIEF-EFD should be preferably used.

Although IIEF questionnaires are an excellent tool for the diagnosis and follow-up of patients with ED, it serves for no purposes during PDU examinations. It is also important to highlight that it does not indicate organicity. Therefore, patients with severe ED from psychogenic etiology might have absolutely normal hemodynamic parameters in PDU.

8.4 Erection Hardness Score (EHS)

Even though the Erection Hardness Score (EHS) is another validated questionnaire, in the context of PDU examinations, it deserves a specific section since it is one of the recommended tools for penile rigidity assessment.

It consists of a single question to quantify erection rigidity: "How would you rate the hardness of your erection?" Possible answers according to the degree of penile tumescence translate into a scoring system is graphically demonstrated in Table 8.2.

Table 8.2 The validated Erection Hardness Score (Ref. [6])

0	*Penis does not enlarge*
1	Penis is larger but not hard
2	Penis is hard, but not enough for penetration
3	Penis is hard enough for penetration but not completely hard
4	Penis is completely hard and fully rigid

Fig. 8.1 Clinical devices to facilitate application of EHS

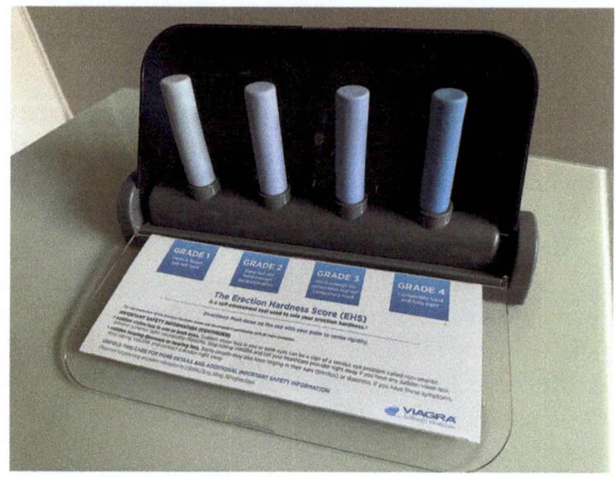

The main benefits of the EHS scale are its simplicity and its ability to clinically assess medical or surgical interventions. It is fact the EHS has a subjective component; however, it provides a clear grading system that has been proved to be very reproducible in clinical practice and directly correlates with the likelihood of satisfactory sexual intercourse. In comparison with most other patient-reported outcomes such as the IIEF, only the EHS concisely assesses erection hardness. The EHS has been widely used since the first clinical trials of phosphodiesterase type 5 inhibitors [7], and it is the most common scale to assess rigidity in the literature of PDU examinations [8].

From the perspective of patients, completing the EHS is uncomplicated and focuses on a clear and relevant outcome. Notably, a global survey of over 3500 men diagnosed with erectile dysfunction revealed that the most crucial factor they look for in an ED treatment is the quality of erections, particularly the ability to achieve and sustain firm erections [6]. In fact, some devices have been manufactured to facilitate understanding of the scale and promote visual and tactile feedback for patients, as shown in Fig. 8.1.

8.4.1 Decimal Scale

The EHS's rationale can be translated into a decimal scale. Although the classic EHS is the most common and broadly used, it is the authors' understanding that the decimal (0–10) erection scale is ideal for the purpose of PDU.

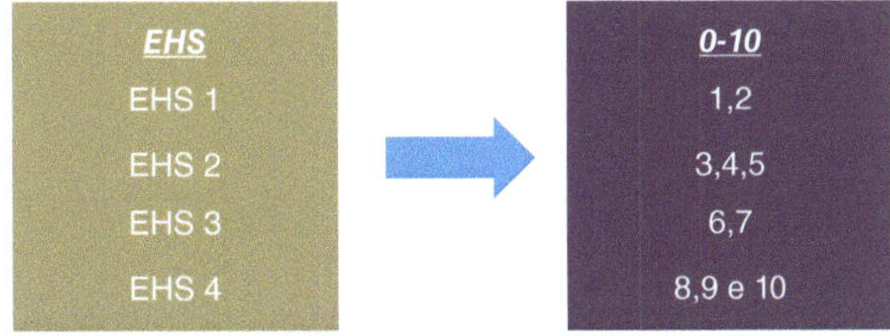

Fig. 8.2 Conversion between EHS and a standard decimal scale for erection rigidity

This decimal scale is an intuitive and easily comprehensible scale. It can be converted into the EHS scale as demonstrated in Fig. 8.2, in which score 6 (or 60%) corresponds to the minimal hardness for penetration (EHS grade 3).

According to the authors' perspective, another important advantage of the decimal scale is adding more granularity to the evaluation. There are some subtleties in erection evaluations that could be easily captured working on a wider-range scale. For example, although erections 3/10 and 5/10 are both considered EHS grade 2, there is a significant difference between these two, since 5/10 sometime varies close to obtaining penetration rigidity.

8.5 Other Measures of Erection Rigidity That Might Be Complementary to PDU

The PDU coupled to a rigidity assessment with the EHS or the decimal scale will provide an overview of penile hemodynamics, which can be a surrogate for radial rigidity; EHS is still based on the examiner's subjective perspective and might eventually lead to conflicting results. Hence, the biggest challenge is to provide an objective measure of axial rigidity. Although studies have revealed good correlation between penile radial and axial rigidity, more direct quantifications of axial rigidity could be beneficial [9].

8.5.1 Digital Rigidometer

As mentioned previously in this chapter, axial rigidity pertains to the erect penis's capacity to resist axial loads and is determined by the mechanical properties of erectile tissue and penile geometry. While radial rigidity has traditionally been used as a proxy for erectile hardness, axial rigidity may be a more appropriate measure, as it is more closely associated with the ability to withstand compressive forces during intercourse [10].

The Digital Inflection Rigidometer (DIR) involves the use of a modified weight scale, which is applied to the erect penis tip in a downward direction during a pharmacologically induced erection, as demonstrated in Fig. 8.3.

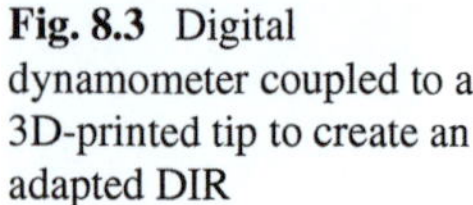

Fig. 8.3 Digital dynamometer coupled to a 3D-printed tip to create an adapted DIR

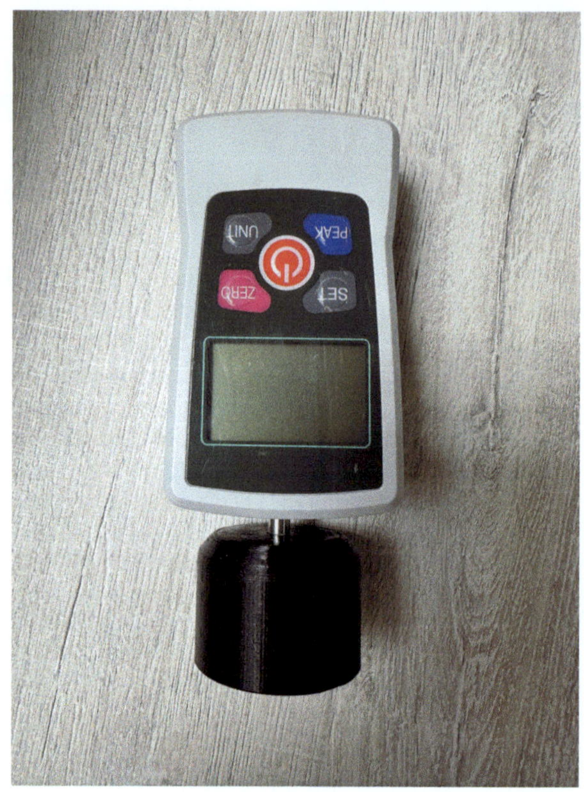

It has been suggested that if the erection hardness can withstand an axial loading force of 1 kg without any bending of the penile shaft, satisfactory penetrable sexual intercourse can be achieved [11]. It can be particularly useful with patients with abnormal penile geometry, commonly found in patients with Peyronie's disease. In such patients, there could be limited axial rigidity as a result of deformities in the penile shaft despite a normal radial rigidity.

Although DIR has been described as promising decades ago, it has not been used in routine practice nowadays, perhaps because of limited availability of devices for such purposes.

It has been considered an easy-to-use instrument for both the patient and providers, without being painful or time-consuming. However, DIR has some limitations, including its inability to measure penile rigidity continuously and its lack of portability for home use [12]. The instrument can only provide static information at a given time during the erection and must be used in the clinical setting. Despite that, it could eventually be used in the setting of PDU, providing additional information of biomechanics of penis while performing penile hemodynamic studies.

8.5.2 *Elastography*

There are promising technology that could be integrated with ultrasound machine devices to provide precise assessments of erectile tissue and penile rigidity. Elastography consists of a noninvasive ultrasound imaging modality for evaluating tissue stiffness [13]. During an erection, the erectile tissue achieves maximum relaxation in order to accommodate blood within the sinusoids. In this phase, the tissue under stretch tends to become stiffer, and it has been proposed that penile rigidity, as measured by density of smooth muscle cells in the corpora cavernosum, may be quantified with the use of elastography [14].

Virtual touch tissue quantification is a possibility to evaluate tissue rigidity using ultrasound technology through an elastography technique known as acoustic radiation force impulse (ARFI) imaging. This method involves measuring shear wave velocity values to detect tissue stiffness. Unlike traditional methods of elastography that require external compression, ARFI imaging uses short-duration acoustic radiation forces to generate shear waves and produce localized displacements in a specific region of interest, allowing for accurate stiffness measurement [15]. A more robust discussion regarding these technologies is provided in a separate chapter of the present book.

8.6 Rigidity-Based vs. Timed-Based Protocols for PDU Hemodynamic Scanning

International standard of practice recommendations for PDU usually suggest that evaluation of hemodynamic parameters be assessed in predefined time points [16]. Multiple time intervals of 5 min are often recommended, up to a total of 30 min of exam duration after intracavernous injection of vasoactive agents. However, there are significant variations in the timing and duration of measurements, with some studies tracking hemodynamic changes for up to 45 min, sometimes with little or no mention of erection rigidity throughout these intervals.

Our suggested approach is to base hemodynamic assessments on the rigidity of the patient's erection rather than predetermined time intervals. We believe that this method is a more precise indicator of complete relaxation of corpus cavernosum smooth muscle. Timed interval scans, such as every 10 min, are not beneficial if the erection rigidity is insufficient. Therefore, while it is crucial for clinicians to provide adequate time for the vasoactive agent to work, the rigidity of the erection should dictate the optimal timing for hemodynamic parameter assessment. Despite that, most studies failed to mention any rigidity assessment, and the report of BQE is only seldom reported in the PDU literature [8].

8.7 How to Assess Penile Rigidity During PDU?

Erection hardness assessment is the basis for redosing protocols of vasoactive agents, so multiple assessments are required during any given PDU examination. All decisions and interpretations will be conducted based on penile rigidity.

In other words, the examiner must get used to constantly reassess erection quality during PDU sessions through visual evaluation and penis palpation. There is usually a learning curve for the examiner to be able to capture such changes in erection rigidity throughout the examination, which are common given the dynamic nature of PDU. Sometimes unilateral abnormalities found in hemodynamic parameters could be a result of adrenalin-mediated loss of erection, which should be promptly recognized.

In order to facilitate this evaluation, we recommend using the 0–10 decimal erection scale (preferably) or the traditional EHS scale. It is important to mention that these two scales are interconvertible.

8.8 Conclusions

An accurate assessment of penile rigidity is key during PDU. According to the chosen rigidity parameter, all decisions and interpretations will be conducted. In other words, the examiner must get used to constantly reassess erection quality during PDU. PDU examiners must become proficient in utilizing the EHS or the decimal scale to perform constant and simultaneous evaluations of erection rigidity. Digital inflexion rigidometer could be eventually added to the PDU procedure to provide a more objective measure of axial rigidity, if available.

References

1. Rohrer GE, Premo H, Lentz AC. Current techniques for the objective measures of erectile hardness. Sex Med Rev. 2022;10(4):648–59.
2. Udelson D. Biomechanics of male erectile function. J R Soc Interface. 2007;4(17):1031–47.
3. Miranda A. Auxetic expansion of the tunica albuginea for penile length and girth restoration without a graft: a translational study. Sex Med. 2021;9(6):100456.
4. Udelson D, Nehra A, Hatzichristou DG, Azadzoi K, Moreland RB, Krane RJ, et al. Engineering analysis of penile hemodynamic and structural-dynamic relationships: part II—clinical implications of penile buckling. Int J Impot Res. 1998;10(1):25–35.
5. Miranda EP, Mulhall JP. International index of erectile function erectile function domain vs the sexually health inventory for men: methodological challenges in the radical prostatectomy population. BJU Int. 2015;115(3):355–6.
6. Goldstein I, Mulhall JP, Bushmakin AG, Cappelleri JC, Hvidsten K, Symonds T. The erection hardness score and its relationship to successful sexual intercourse. J Sex Med. 2008;5(10):2374–80.

7. Mulhall JP, Goldstein I, Bushmakin AG, Cappelleri JC, Hvidsten K. Validation of the erection hardness score. J Sex Med. 2007;4(6):1626–34.
8. Nascimento B, Miranda EP, Terrier JE, Carneiro F, Mulhall JP. A critical analysis of methodology pitfalls in duplex Doppler ultrasound in the evaluation of patients with erectile dysfunction: technical and interpretation deficiencies. J Sex Med. 2020;17(8):1416–22.
9. Mizuno I, Komiya A, Watanabe A, Fuse H. Importance of axial penile rigidity in objective evaluation of erection quality in patients with erectile dysfunction—comparison with radial rigidity. Urol Int. 2010;84(2):194–7.
10. Wilson SK, Cleves MA, Delk JR 2nd. Long-term follow-up of treatment for Peyronie's disease: modeling the penis over an inflatable penile prosthesis. J Urol. 2001;165(3):825–9.
11. Rosselló BM. Digital inflection rigidometry in the study of erectile dysfunction. A new technique. Arch Esp Urol. 1996;49(3):221–7.
12. Mizuno I, Fuse H, Fujiuchi Y, Nakagawa O, Akashi T. Comparative study between audiovisual sexual stimulation test and nocturnal penile tumescence test using RigiScan plus in the evaluation of erectile dysfunction. Urol Int. 2004;72(3):221–4.
13. Arda K, Ciledag N, Aktas E, Arıbas BK, Köse K. Quantitative assessment of normal soft-tissue elasticity using shear-wave ultrasound elastography. Am J Roentgenol. 2011;197(3):532–6.
14. Inci E, Turkay R, Nalbant MO, Yenice MG, Tugcu V. The value of shear wave elastography in the quantification of corpus cavernosum penis rigidity and its alteration with age. Eur J Radiol. 2017;89:106–10.
15. Hsiao W, Bennett N, Guhring P, Narus J, Mulhall JP. Satisfaction profiles in men using intracavernosal injection therapy. J Sex Med. 2011;8(2):512–7.
16. Sikka SC, Hellstrom WJ, Brock G, Morales AM. Standardization of vascular assessment of erectile dysfunction: standard operating procedures for duplex ultrasound. J Sex Med. 2013;10(1):120–9.

Chapter 9
Audiovisual Sexual Stimulation During Hemodynamic Evaluation of the Penis

9.1   Introduction

Even before the use of penile Doppler ultrasound (PDU) with intracavernous injection of vasoactive agents in the evaluation of erectile dysfunction (ED), audiovisual sexual stimulation (AVSS) was already performed. As previously discussed in Chap. 1, nocturnal penile tumescence (NPT) testing was once the gold standard to ED evaluation. It was thought to be useful in distinguishing psychogenic from organic ED, as it was used to obtain an accurate indication of the quantity and quality of erections that normally occur during the alpha phase of the sleep. In fact, identification of psychogenic ED has always been a concern to clinicians and researchers, who have always tried to distinguish it from organic ED. Then, NPT started to be replaced by penile plethysmography (PP) in awake individuals. Pulse of the dorsal penile artery and changes in penile circumference were measured during erotic film stimuli as showed in Fig. 9.1 [1].

Sexually induced erections are distinct from sleep erections. Sexually generated erections are a combination of erotic and reflex erection activity, whereas the mechanism underlying the initiation and maintenance of sleep erections remains unexplained. The primary distinction between sleep and sexually induced erections is neurological, since both erections involve the identical penile and vascular structural components [2]. A complex set of cortical and subcortical brain regions, including the Anterior and Middle Cingulate Cortex, the Insula, the Claustrum, and the Hypothalamus, have been described in a number of neuroimaging studies conducted in healthy volunteers over the last decades using visual sexual stimulation [3]. In 1980, Kockott et al. pioneered the use of erotic movies in the evaluation of sexual disorders [4]. They studied penile response by erotic film stimuli in men with ED in comparison to a control group of men without ED. Variations in blood pressure, penile erection duration, latency, and amplitude were assessed in 42

E. d. P. Miranda, F. Carneiro, *Penile Color Duplex-Doppler Ultrasound in Erectile Dysfunction Diagnosis and Management*,
https://doi.org/10.1007/978-3-031-55649-4_9

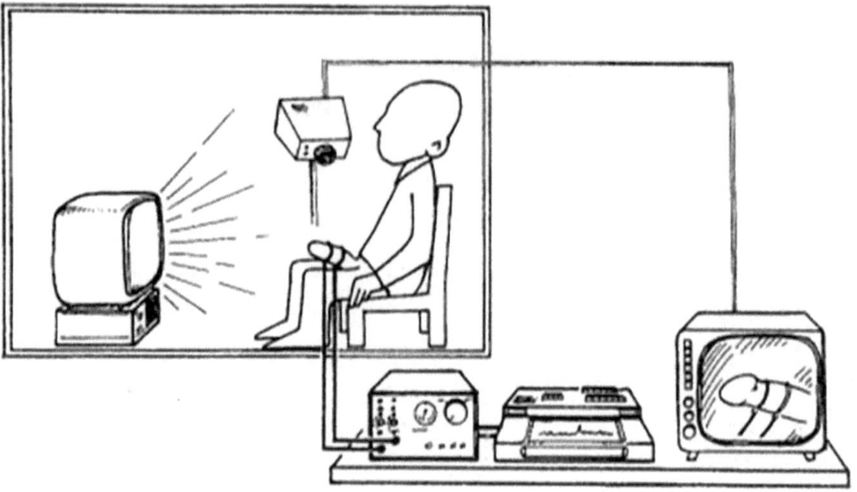

Fig. 9.1 Penile pletismography [1]. Erection monitored while patient is isolated in front of a video monitor with erotic film

individuals, and the group of men with ED had considerably worse parameters. After that, other investigators have also advocated the use of AVSS [5, 6], as it may enhance parasympathetic tone by inhibiting sympathetic tone, which leads to a better erection than with a vasoactive agent injection alone [7, 8].

9.2   Audiovisual Sexual Stimulation and Penile Doppler Ultrasound

In order to obtain consistent result in penile hemodynamic evaluation with PDU, it is mandatory to have complete smooth muscle relaxation (CSMR) of the erectile tissue. This is crucial to avoid false positive results [9]. A mistaken diagnosis of arterial insufficiency (AI) and/or corporal venous occlusive disorder (CVOD) may result from excessive sympathetic discharge as it prevents complete CMSR in response to vasoactive drugs [10, 11]. From all possible strategies to allow CSMR, redosing of intracavernous vasodilators was introduced as a pivotal strategy [11]. However, de Meyer and Thibo [12] suggested that occasionally redosing alone was not sufficient to induce CSMR in their prospective study measuring the effect of a redosing protocol on intracavernous pressure.

In this scenario, AVSS has also been described as a means to increase sexual arousal, which could potentially lead to lower rates of false diagnoses on PDU. Katlowitz et al. reported that the majority of men in their sample of 25 patients had improved penile hemodynamic parameters on PDU examination following

AVSS [7]. It seems reasonable to infer that the whole environment of PDU to assess erectile function of men with ED is stressful, and AVSS can be considered a tool to simulate an environment closer to the bedroom scenario. From a biological perspective, it is thought that AVSS leads to an increase in parasympathetic output, resulting in better vasodilation and relaxation of the corpora cavernosa and consequently in a more rigid erection than with ICI alone [7, 8].

Montorsi et al. [13] compared the redosing technique versus ICI plus AVSS and reported 87% maximum rigidity with vasoactive injection and AVSS against 47% with up to 1 redosing of alprostadil 10mcg. Similar findings were reported by Pescatori et al. [14], who demonstrated that 80% of the patients with AVSS vs. 33% of the patients without AVSS achieved CSMR after the first ICI. The same study also suggested that AVSS could reduce the need of redosing, possibly reducing the chance of prolonged erections and/or priapism. Interestingly, in this study some non-responders to redosing did still have complete CSMR when AVSS was added.

9.3   Lessons from a Prospective Study

At our institution, we have also conducted a prospective study to evaluate AVSS during PDU tests [15]. The study's objective was to assess the impact of the AVSS during PDU in ED patients, looking at how this strategy affected hemodynamic parameters and final diagnosis. Men who were heterosexual and older than 18 who had an ED diagnosis were invited to participate. Partnered sexual activity, a history of ED for at least 6 months, and a self-reported poor response to phosphodiesterase type 5 inhibitors were the inclusion criteria. Patients who had previously undergone PDU studies or who were previously or currently using ICI as an ED therapy were excluded. A total of 40 patients were included and each patient underwent 2 PDU examinations with and without AVSS 7 days apart from each other with a fixed dose of ICI containing 20 mcg of alprostadil. To avoid sequential bias and minimize the accommodation effect of repeat testing in PDU, sessions were randomized so that half of the patients had AVSS on the first examination and the other half on the second.

There was a considerable rise in the cavernous artery diameters after ICI in all sessions, but it was more obvious with AVSS scanning, regardless of the session order and laterality. End diastolic velocity (EDV) and resistance index (RI) had better values with AVSS regardless the session order. Those parameters are an indirect way to measure corporal smooth muscle relaxation. The proportion of patients whose final PDU diagnosis was altered due to AVSS intervention was 4/40 (10%, 95% confidence interval [CI]: 2.8–23.7%). Three of the 12 patients diagnosed with CVOD by the PDU without AVSS were considered normal by PDU with AVSS (25.0%, 95% CI: 5.5–87.2%). Among the 4 patients diagnosed with AI by the first PDU without AVSS, one became normal by the second PDU with AVSS (25.0%,

95% confidence interval [CI]: 0.6–80.6%).Out of 28 patients with normal PDU, 50% had negative EDV without AVSS compared to 67.9% with AVSS ($P = 0.3$). When we split those numbers up by session, we discovered that in the second session, 88.2% of patients with AVSS and 72.7% of patients without AVSS had zero or negative EDVs. In the second session, when we isolated negative EDV, we discovered 76.5% vs. 36.4% of the patients with AVSS and without AVSS, respectively.

Patients who performed the second session without AVSS had higher PSV values, reinforcing the idea that patient accommodation may have an impact on repeat PDU parameters. The erectile tissue relaxation response may not be fully attained even in the presence of AVSS when a patient undergoes PDU investigations for the first time because of an elevated adrenergic tone brought on by apprehension and worry. This is a prevalent source of bias in the PDU research; as such design may unintentionally overestimate the impact of any given intervention. The randomized use of AVSS in various session orders was pertinent addition to the literature, as only one previous study has had a similar design to prevent sequential bias [5].

Additionally, we showed that AVSS led to a higher rise in cavernous artery diameters. Although it is not the best metric to show adequate blood flow to the penis, it could be used as a substitute marker for cavernosal artery vasodilation in response to a similar dose of a vasoactive drug.

Theoretically, improving EDV and RI values would be the most pertinent effect of adding AVSS in the PDU practice because decreased smooth muscle relaxation is more likely to have an impact on intracavernous pressure regardless of PSVs.

Kuo et al. [5] discovered considerably superior penile hemodynamic parameters by combining AVSS and ICI. Pescatori et al. [14] confirmed that patients stimulated with AVSS were at least twice as likely to have normal PSVs, and they also observed similar findings. Better EDV values were also seen with AVSS by Tang et al. [6], but in this study, AVSS sessions were always repeated.

In the PDU session with AVSS, a greater percentage of men had negative EDVs (67.9% vs. 50%). Similar to the proportions of zero or negative EDVs, the second session with the AVSS had a greater absolute value than the second session without the AVSS (88.2% vs. 72.7%).

It is noteworthy to note that even in individuals with EDs that were severe, we discovered negative EDVs and high RI values. Even men with moderate or severe ED may be affected by psychogenic factors and have normal Doppler parameters.

The ability of AVSS to alter PDU diagnosis was the most important finding of our research. We have found 4 patients (25%) had a normal PDU evaluation with ICI plus AVSS, out of the 16 patients with aberrant hemodynamics according to PDU with ICI alone (12 with CVOD and 4 with AI). In a similar vein, Kuo et al. [5] observed that the addition of AVSS resulted in 12% diagnostic change across the board and 18% altered PDU studies. These findings might improve the patient's prognosis because an abnormal PDU typically necessitates more intrusive treatments.

9.4 Recommendations of AVSS

After discussing multiple potential benefits of AVSS, it is the authors' recommendation to include AVSS in the routine of penile hemodynamic studies. There are no reported side effects of short time use of this strategy during PDU. However, it is important to highlight that it might be a sensitive issue in some circumstances and PDU examiners must be careful when offering in-office AVSS.

First, there might be religious restrictions to pornography consumption or masturbation. So, it is important to capture some of these patient's characteristics during initial sexual history. Permission should always be obtained prior to AVSS, and it is important to explain the importance of mimicking a sexual scenario to obtain CSMR and the best possible outcome. An important argument is that AVSS will also decrease the need for redosing and, therefore, the incidence of potential complications such as prolonged erections and priapism.

Another important aspect that should be inquired previously is sexual orientation and/or preferences. Therefore, it is important to have a variety of options for diverse patients and not only heterosexual content. Beware that with the advent of smartphones, some patients might prefer to use their own collection or to visit an online website of preference. Finally, it is important to be cautious about AVSS content, avoiding violence or other unpleasant depicts of sexual activity that might have the opposite effect in some patients. Having a full range of options that any patient can browse through is perhaps the ideal scenario.

9.5 Conclusion

AVSS has been characterized in the literature as beneficial in the evaluation of ED because it places the patient in a more realistic sexual situation and lowers the adrenergic tone, resulting in a higher rate of CSMR during PDU. The combination of ICI and AVSS may be an even more effective erectogenic strategy than high doses of ICI alone in the PDU setting. This helpful tool improves PDU accuracy and may be crucial for a precise diagnosis. It is the authors' recommendation that AVSS be routinely offered to patients during PDU.

References

1. Opsomer R-J, Wese F-X, Van Cangh P. Visual sexual stimulation plethysmooraphy: complementary test to nocturnal penile plethysmooraphy. Urology. 1990;35(6):504–7.
2. Cera N, Di Pierro ED, Ferretti A, Tartaro A, Romani GL, Perrucci MG. Brain networks during free viewing of complex erotic movie: new insights on psychogenic erectile dysfunction. PLoS One. 2014;9(8):e105336.

3. Stoleru S, Gregoire M-C, Gerard D, Decety J, Lafarge E, Cinotti L, et al. Neuroanatomical correlates of visually evoked sexual arousal in human males. Arch Sex Behav. 1999;28(1):1–21.
4. Kockott G, Feil W, Ferstl R, Aldenhoff J, Besinger U. Psychophysiological aspects of male sexual inadequacy: results of an experimental study. Arch Sex Behav. 1980;9(6):477–93.
5. Kuo YC, Liu SP, Chen JH, Chang HC, Tsai VF, Hsieh JT. Feasability of a novel audio-video sexual stimulation system: an adjunct to the use of penile duplex Doppler ultrasonography for the investigation of erectile dysfunction. J Sex Med. 2010;7(12):3979–83.
6. Tang J, Tang Y, Dai Y, Lu L, Jiang X. The use of intracavernous injection and audiovisual sexual stimulation during real-time pharmacopenile Doppler ultrasonography in vasculogenic erectile dysfunction. Urol Int. 2013;90(4):460–4.
7. Katlowitz NM, Albano GJT, Morales P, Golimbu M. Potentiation of drug-induced erection with audiovisual sexual stimulation. Urology. 1993;41(5):431–4.
8. Montorsi F, Guazzoni G, Barbeiri L, Ferini-Strambi L, Iannaccone S, Calori G, et al. Genital plus audiovisual sexual stimulation following intracavernous vasoactive injection versus redosing for erectile dysfunction—results of a prospective study. J Urol. 1998;159(1):113–5.
9. Saenz de Tejada I, Moroukian P, Tessier J, Kim J, Goldstein I, Frohrib D. Trabecular smooth muscle modulates the capacitor function of the penis. Studies on a rabbit model. Am J Physiol. 1991;260(5):H1590–5.
10. Aversa A, Rocchietti-March M, Caprio M, Giannini D, Isidori A, Fabbri A. Anxiety-induced failure in erectile response to intracorporeal prostaglandin-E1 in non-organic male impotence: a new diagnostic approach. Int J Androl. 1996;19(5):307–13.
11. Hatzichristou DG, De Tejada IS, Kupferman S, Namburi S, Pescatori ES, Udelson D, et al. In vivo assessment of trabecular smooth muscle tone, its application in pharmaco-cavernosometry and analysis of intracavernous pressure determinants. J Urol. 1995;153(4):1126–35.
12. de Meyer J-M, Thibo P. The effect of re-dosing of vasodilators on the intracavernosal pressure and on the penile rigidity. Eur Urol. 1998;33(3):293–7.
13. Montorsi F, Guazzoni G, Barbieri L, Galli L, Rigatti P, Pizzini G, et al. The effect of intracorporeal injection plus genital and audiovisual sexual stimulation versus second injection on penile color Doppler sonography parameters. J Urol. 1996;155(2):536–40.
14. Pescatori E, Silingardi V, Galeazzi GM, Rigatelli M, Ranzi A, Artibani W. Audiovisual sexual stimulation by virtual glasses is effective in inducing complete cavernosal smooth muscle relaxation: a pharmacocavernosometric study. Int J Impot Res. 2000;12(2):83.
15. Carneiro F, Nascimento B, Miranda EP, Cury J, Cerri GG, Chammas MC. Audiovisual sexual stimulation improves diagnostic accuracy of penile doppler ultrasound in patients with erectile dysfunction. J Sex Med. 2020;17(2):249–56.

Chapter 10
Erection Reversal Protocols and Management of Prolonged Erections

10.1 Introduction

One of the main principles of penile hemodynamics studies with an induced erection is that no patient may be discharged with a rigid erection. Prolonged erections and priapism are undoubtedly the most feared complications of intracavernous injections of vasoactive injection because it might lead to irreversible compromise of erectile tissue. Because of its time-dependent and progressive nature, priapism is a situation that both urologists and radiologists that perform PDU must have adequate skills to manage. Therefore, a fundamental part of penile Doppler ultrasound (PDU) examinations is to reassess erection rigidity in a predetermined period of time and proceed with erection reversal or early penile aspiration whenever necessary. If performed correctly, this strategy will prevent entirely the risk of priapism, since reevaluation and reversal of erection should occur way before 4 h. In this chapter, the most relevant nuances of erection reversal will be discussed, as detumescence protocols are as important as those for erection induction. Priapism related to sickle cell disease (SCD) and other hematological conditions usually have a different pathophysiology and are beyond the scope of the present discussion, though many references and knowledge acquired in this field are derived from such conditions.

10.2 Physiology of the Flaccid Penis

When the smooth muscle is contracted, the penis remains in a flaccid state. The smooth muscle contraction is regulated by a combination of adrenergic control from noradrenaline, intrinsic myogenic control and endothelium-derived contracting factors such as prostaglandin and endothelins [1]. Noradrenaline signaling mainly

E. d. P. Miranda, F. Carneiro, *Penile Color Duplex-Doppler Ultrasound in
Erectile Dysfunction Diagnosis and Management*,
https://doi.org/10.1007/978-3-031-55649-4_10

regulates calcium influx into cells, which binds to calmodulin and facilitating the formation of the calmodulin–myosin light chain kinase (MLCK) complex. This leads to the phosphorylation of MLC, resulting in smooth muscle contraction and a flaccid penis. Noradrenaline signaling also inhibits adenylyl cyclase (AC) and modulates the RHO-associated protein kinase (ROCK) pathway, which increases the sensitivity of MLC to calcium [2, 3].

When the smooth muscle is contracted, inflow of blood through the cavernous artery is minimal, and blood outflows freely through the subtunical venules. Basically, stimulation of the adrenergic pathway is the most important step in detumescence protocols.

10.3   Definitions of Prolonged Erection and Priapism

Priapism is the most severe adverse event following intracavernous (IC) injections of vasoactive agents characterized by an erection lasting over 4 h. Prolonged erections are defined as an erection with more than 2 h of duration [4, 5]. Ischemic priapism is defined by rigid corpora, minimal or no cavernous blood inflow, and complete occlusion of venous outflow. Interestingly, the glans and corpus spongiosum may be flaccid or partially engorged but are usually not rigid. Corporal nociceptors are activated by the high acidity contained within the compartment, leading to the presence of pain, which is usually present. Persistent and progressive pain may be considered an early sign that an induced erection is leading to an ischemic event and that will probably require intervention in the PDU setting.

It is important to make a distinction from nonischemic priapism that is usually secondary to traumatic arterial shunt that overflow the corpora with oxygenated blood, which is not a medical emergency and is also known as high-flow priapism. Nonischemic priapism following IC injections leading to inadvertent lesions of cavernosal or helicine arteries has never been reported, though theoretically possible.

10.4   Physiopathology of Ischemic Priapism

Early recognition and management of priapism cases are essential, as delays to induce detumescence might result in irreversible damage. Priapism creates an oxygen-deprived environment in the penis due to the stagnant blood flow in the cavernous bodies, leading to the accumulation of CO_2 levels and eventual tissue damage. This damage triggers necrosis and extensive inflammation, cavernous thrombosis, and smooth muscle necrosis, ultimately replacing healthy tissue with fibrotic scar tissue. As a result, severe erectile dysfunction (ED) may develop due to these irreversible changes [6].

Time is of utmost importance in terms of tissue damage after priapism. According to the literature on patients with SCD, if ischemic priapism is reversed within 24 h, there is usually a recovery of erectile function in approximately 50% of patients, while duration of more than 36 h uniformly results in complete necrosis of the erectile tissue. An ischemic time of 12–24 h lead to variable outcomes, and apparently patients with priapism following IC injections of vasoactive agents tend to have a more favorable prognosis. Also, as opposed to priapism secondary to SCD, initial treatment with local measures and injection of reversal agents can achieve detumescence in the vast majority of cases, decreasing the need for invasive procedures or surgery as a first-line therapy alternative [7].

10.5 Epidemiology

The incidence of prolonged erection or ischemic priapism following diagnostic penile injection of vasoactive agents in the office is reported to vary between 1.3 and 5.3% [8, 9]. Moreover, these numbers might vary according to the etiology or clinical aspects of ED, being considerably higher in younger men, in patients with neurogenic or psychogenic ED, and in those reported recreational use without proper medical supervision [4]. However, it is the authors' understanding that priapism episodes following PDU examination should be nonexistent, since it is the examiners responsibility to make sure the penis has achieved a safe state of detumescence prior to patient discharge.

10.6 Detumescence Strategies

As already mentioned in this chapter, prevention of prolonged erections is perhaps the most important step in any given PDU clinic. First, redosing strategies for inducing an erection should be carefully performed to avoid unnecessary high dosage of IC agents, in which redosing should be adjusted according to penile rigidity. Also, it is important to have a relaxant environment and trained personnel to minimize patient anxiety. Audiovisual and manual stimulation is also encouraged in order to minimize the need for repeat IC injections [10].

We recommend that the physician and/or the medical team combined devote at least 1–1.5 h in the schedule for each patient who is performing PDU examinations. The exact time of the first IC injection should be recorded, and predetermined reassessments of penile rigidity should be performed, minimizing delay on IC injection of reversal agents whenever necessary. Keep in mind that aspiration is very rarely required, but adequate instruments for such procedure should be always readily available.

10.6.1   Non-pharmacological Interventions and Oral Medications

Historically, low complexity interventions have been suggested for patients with prolonged erections such as ejaculation, ice packs, cold baths, cold-water enemas, voiding, and exercise. The rationales behind these strategies consisted basically to induce contraction of the cavernous smooth muscle, aiding in the detumescence process. However, there is a lack of evidence reporting the effectiveness of such measures.

Oral medications with sympathetic action such as etilefrine, pseudoephedrine, phenylpropanolamine, and terbutaline have been recommended for the same purpose. These medications have demonstrated efficacy rates in reverting prolonged erections of less than 4 h of 28–42% [11, 12]. However, to date these oral agents are not recommended in the management of acute ischemic priapism >4 h.

While some these strategies could be tried in the setting of long-term IC therapy prior to or on the way to a medical facility, or even while the patient waits successive reevaluations during PDU with no harm or delay to the injection of reversal agents, these should not be considered a primary strategy for achieving detumescence.

10.6.2   Intracavernous Sympathomimetic Agents

Sympathomimetic amines have been utilized for the management of acute priapism attacks since 1986. The substances induce rapid cavernous smooth muscle contraction, aiming to generate immediate detumescence of the penis. The most common representatives of this class of medication and their specific action in adrenoreceptors are demonstrated in Table 10.1.

There is a lack of comparative trials and dosage-tolerating studies to report on the use of sympathomimetic agents in managing priapism. The efficacy of these agents varies in the literature, ranging from 43 to 81%, with reported time-dependent efficacies for each agent. Additionally, the availability of adrenergic agents worldwide varies substantially. However, the reversal of priapism has been effectively documented with diluted injections of phenylephrine, etilefrine, epinephrine, ephedrine, or metaraminol.

Table 10.1 List of the most common sympathomimetic agents and adrenoreceptor activity

Drug	$\alpha 1$	$\alpha 2$	$\beta 1$	$\beta 2$
Epinephrine	++	++	+++	+++
Norepinephrine	+++	+++	++	+
Phenylephrine	++	0	0	0
Etilefrine	++	0	+	0
Metaraminol	++	0	+	0
Ephedrine	++	+	+	+

Some sympathomimetic drugs are activators of both alpha and beta adrenergic receptors. Ideally, drugs with a more specific action on alpha1 receptor should be preferably given, to avoid cardiac side effects. To ensure patient safety, physicians must closely monitor patients for subjective cardiovascular complaints and objective findings that are consistent with known adverse effects such as headache, chest discomfort, dizziness, acute hypertension, reflex bradycardia, tachycardia, palpitations, and cardiac arrhythmia. It is recommended to conduct blood pressure monitoring if repeated dosing of sympathomimetic agents is given. In patients with significant cardiovascular risks or extremes of age, electrocardiogram monitoring is also advisable.

10.6.2.1 Phenylephrine

Phenylephrine is a sympathomimetic drug with the most selective alpha1 adrenergic receptor selectivity, supposedly with less ionotropic and chronotropic cardiac effects, which leads to a more favorable side-effect profile [13]. Therefore, it is the agent of choice for intracavernous management of ischemic priapism whenever available [14].

Phenylephrine is usually diluted in normal saline with a concentration of 100–500 µg/mL and given in 1 mL dosages every 3–5 min. Although no recommendations can be made about maximum safe dosing, hypertensive stroke with subarachnoid hemorrhage has been reported as a complication of cumulative dosing of 2 mg. Therefore, dosing should be intermittent over the course of an hour with an injection every 5–10 min to a maximum dosage of 1 mg. This will permit up to ten separate injections of 0.5 mL (100 µg each) or five separate injections of 1 mL [4].

10.6.2.2 Etilefrine

Etilefrine is an alpha1-selective agonist with minor beta1 activity. When used as an IC injection, it has minimal cardiovascular adverse effects with short-term efficacy and safety being reported by several groups [15, 16]. Although phenylephrine is the sympathomimetic drug of choice according to the most recent AUA guidelines, many regions outside the United States have used etilefrine in a similar fashion because of availability issues [7]. For example, in Brazil phenylephrine is only available for hospital use, so most PDU clinics have to use etilefrine as their primary agent.

Classically, it may be diluted in normal saline, and the intracavernous dosage of etilefrine 1–4 mg per injection is recommended in order to achieve detumescence. The onset of action of etilefrine is relatively rapid, typically within 5–15 min after injection. One of the advantages of etilefrine is its relatively short duration of action in comparison to phenylephrine (30 min vs. 1–2 h), which brings less concerns regarding cumulative dosage of multiple injections [17].

10.6.2.3   Epinephrine

Epinephrine may be used in detumescence protocols, although it is not considered an ideal initial option. Because of its significant cardiovascular effects, it might be a dangerous agent with lethal outcomes after dosing errors. There is a case report of a 16-year-old boy who received 4 mL intracavernous injection of undiluted 1:1000 (1 mg/mL) epinephrine solution and had a cardiac arrest. It is possible that epinephrine is the only available reversal agent in some emergency department cases of priapism. In this case, an ideal dilution would be 1:1,000,000 (1 mg/mL vial to 1 L saline or 0.001 mg/mL). The authors recommend extreme caution when using epinephrine, which is eventually reserved for concomitant aspiration procedures in an intent of providing a more copious washing of the corpora cavernosa usually for refractory and dramatic cases of priapism. This should not be the case for prolonged erection following PDU examinations.

10.6.2.4   Other Amines

There are other sympathomimetic amines with alpha-adrenergic agonist effects that might be used to induce contraction of penile smooth muscle to generate detumescence in the context of PDU. These other agents such as metaraminol and ephedrine are also an option that have been demonstrated to be safe and effective, though the evidence to support their use is more limited. However, we understand that they might be the most acceptable options in certain circumstances. It is important to mention that all agents used in the erection reversal are also used in hospital settings because they are also useful for their vasopressor effects in anesthesia and intensive care units. If required, careful revision of the pharmacological properties of these drugs is warranted prior to using them in clinical practice.

For example, the recommended starting dose of metaraminol for the treatment of priapism is typically around 0.5–1 mg, which can be increased in increments of 0.5–1 mg if needed. The maximum dose of metaraminol used for priapism is typically around 5 mg, although the specific dose used may vary depending on the individual patient and their response to the medication.

10.6.2.5   In-Office Aspiration Procedures

First of all, it is important to mention that aspirations will very rarely be required if detumescence protocols are strictly followed. However, it is fundamental that the examiner be prepared for this specific moment with no unnecessary delays. Having said that, it is very important that the examiner himself or someone from the team properly trained in penile aspiration procedures always be available during PDU schedules. If pre-established protocols are defined, these situations tend not to be dramatic.

It is the authors' understanding that the PDU clinics should be readily equipped for performing penile aspirations whenever needed. Having to transfer the patient to the emergency department in different locations will eventually delay the procedure and worsen the overall traumatic experience to the patient.

Initial preparation for any given aspiration technique should include administration of a dorsal nerve block with appropriate local anesthetic agent (Fig. 10.1). After proper anesthesia, a large-gauge needle (19 gauge or higher) is placed into the corpora. Although it is most commonly recommended inserting the needle in the lateral aspect of the penis, the authors of this book prefer a transglandular approach, as demonstrated in Fig. 10.2. Lateral punctures in the fully rigid penis increase the risk of blood extravasation and hematoma formation within Bucks fascia, which might compress the puncture site and contribute to recurrence of priapism. On the other

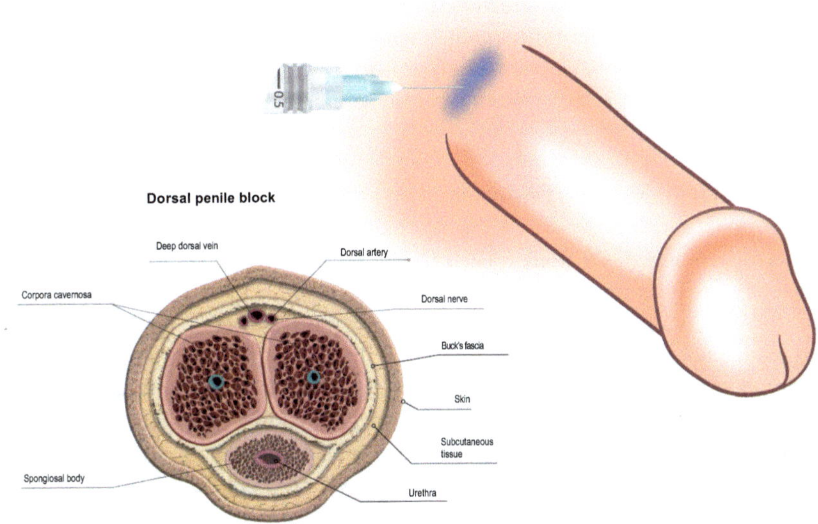

Fig. 10.1 Penile block technique

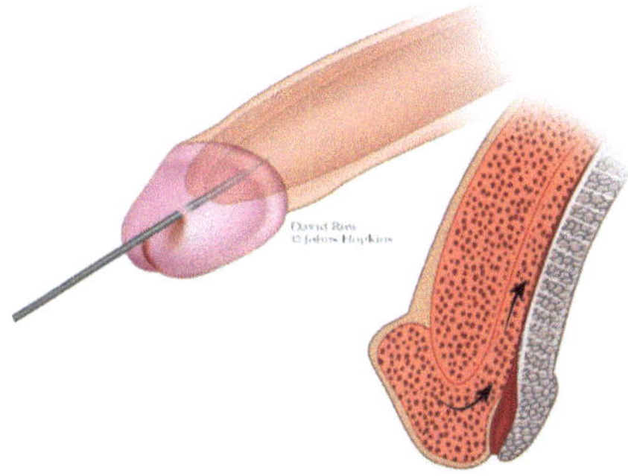

Fig. 10.2 Schematic demonstration of an initial transglandular approach to penile aspiration during prolonged erections

hand, a transglandular approach after penile block is usually painless, allows immediate detumescence, and does not predispose to hematoma formation. In fact, this approach will favor a temporary distal shunt, aiding in a quick, safe, and effective procedure. After removing the needle, eventual blood extravasation will help further in draining the blood and not lead to hematoma formation. Suturing of the puncture in the glans penis is usually not necessary. This technique is a recommendation according to the authors' preference, although others are also very efficient. The most important aspect is that someone in PDU team must be ready at all times to perform a safe and effective procedure for penile aspiration.

Aspiration of small volumes of blood in the scenario of short-term prolonged erections following PDU examinations usually leads to fast detumescence and almost instantaneous restoration of the corporal environment with oxygenated blood, which is required for effective smooth muscle contraction in response to sympathomimetic drugs. The entire process results in a significant reduction of intracavernous pressure, provides pain relief, and improves the corporal environment by removing blood that is deprived of oxygen, acidic, and high in carbon dioxide.

10.6.2.6 Detumescence Protocols

Priapism/prolonged erections related to in-office erectile function testing for PDU is usually easily reversed in most cases because the time of ischemia is considerably short. We recommend start reversing diagnostic erections after 1 h. Though it might not seem a considerable amount of time for the pathophysiology of priapism, it has been reported that the process of smooth muscle cell edema may start early in cases of very high intracavernous pressure. It is also a known fact that these cells with edema and in poor oxygenated environments tend to have an inadequate response to sympathomimetics, proving that starting reversal protocols at 1 h might be beneficial [4]. Also, shorter assessment intervals avoid excessive discharging time in each patients, which makes it easier to accommodate more exams in any given working schedule. Since discharging patients without reassessment is not an option, and waiting up to 4 h in with every single patient is not cost effective, it is our understanding that 1 h since first injection for the erection inducing protocol is generally ideal for rigidity reassessment.

The recommend detumescence protocol is found in Table 10.2. We recommend phenylephrine or etilefrine as drugs of choice since these are the ones with the most

Table 10.2 Step-by-step recommendation of a highly effective detumescence protocol

Detumescence protocol
1. Start reversing diagnostic erections after 1 h of inducing an erection
2. Phenylephrine in 1000 µg/mL or etilefrine in 10 mg/mL should be preferably used with aliquots of: phenylephrine 200–300 µg, or etilefrine 5–10 mg
3. Try to reach maximum dose within 3 doses after 10 min intervals
4. In non-responsive patients, fixed rigid erection proceed directly to in-office penile aspiration following penile dorsal nerve block

specificity for adrenergic alpha1 receptor activity and with the highest availability globally. Initial doses of phenylephrine 200–300 µg and etilefrine 5–10 mg using an ultrafine needle and 1 mL syringe are recommended. The dilution preferences are phenylephrine in 1000 µg/mL and etilefrine in 10 mg/mL. It is also our routine to limit the maximal number of injection to 3 after 10 min intervals, which can be more easily obtained with more concentrated preparations. Such of this experience comes from studies in hypotensive subjects demonstrating that etilefrine 5–10 mg may be given to adults by slow intravenous injection during anesthetic procedures. However, caution is always recommended, especially for those who are in their learning curve. It is perfectly understandable and reasonable to allow more than three injections and more time with each patient until detumescence is obtained whenever required.

Here it is important to remind the principle of the closed compartment within the corpora during an erection. While the veno-occlusive mechanism is functioning, there is minimal or no circulation of blood. Therefore, injection of vasoconstriction agents in this microenvironment does not reach systemic circulation right away, which tends to decrease systemic side effects. It is important to inform patients about the possible negative implications of phenylephrine or etilefrine administration, which may include symptoms such as headache, palpitations, and dizziness. In fact, the onset of these systemic side effects usually indicates initial detumescence of the penis.

The maximal dose recommended is up to 1000 µg of phenylephrine and 30 mg of etilefrine, which are usually effective without significant hypertension/reflex bradycardia in a healthy normotensive adult. Moreover, it is prudent for patients undergoing repeated sympathomimetic injections to be under sequential blood pressure monitoring.

If the patient remains with a fixed rigid erection, which appears to not have been responding at all to additional injections of vasopressors, then examiners should proceed directly to penile aspiration. In the authors' experience, up to 70% may be reversed after the first injection of medium-to-high concentrations of sympathomimetic agents, around 25% will require a second injection, and up to 5% will require the third one. These numbers indicate that less than 0.3% will proceed to aspiration if all the principles mentioned above were followed.

10.7 Conclusions

One of the most important issues in the management of priapism/prolonged erection is prevention, avoiding excessive redosing of vasoactive agents during erection-induction. No patient should be discharged if presenting a penetration-rigid erection following PDU examination. A detumescence protocol should be started ideally after 1 h of primary induction of the erection and should ideally include sequential injection of intracavernous sympathomimetic agents. Although different options of reversal agents are possible, phenylephrine or etilefrine should be preferably used.

If a fixed erection persists despite sympathomimetic injections, we recommend proceeding to in-office cavernosal aspiration. If these recommended are strictly followed, aspiration procedures will be required very rarely. However, it does not exempt the examiners from the responsibility to have adequate training and infrastructure for such a type of intervention.

References

1. Yafi FA, Jenkins L, Albersen M, Corona G, Isidori AM, Goldfarb S, et al. Erectile dysfunction. Nat Rev Dis Primers. 2016;2:16003.
2. Lue TF. Erectile dysfunction. N Engl J Med. 2000;342(24):1802–13.
3. Saenz de Tejada I, Kim N, Lagan I, Krane RJ, Goldstein I. Regulation of adrenergic activity in penile corpus cavernosum. J Urol. 1989;142(4):1117–21.
4. Ericson C, Baird B, Broderick GA. Management of priapism: 2021 update. Urol Clin North Am. 2021;48(4):565–76.
5. Virag R, Bachir D, Lee K, Galacteros F. Preventive treatment of priapism in sickle cell disease with oral and self-administered intracavernous injection of etilefrine. Urology. 1996;47(5):777–81; discussion 81.
6. Broderick GA, Kadioglu A, Bivalacqua TJ, Ghanem H, Nehra A, Shamloul R. Priapism: pathogenesis, epidemiology, and management. J Sex Med. 2010;7(1 Pt 2):476–500.
7. Saffon Cuartas JP, Sandoval-Salinas C, Martínez JM, Corredor HA. Treatment of priapism secondary to drugs for erectile dysfunction. Adv Urol. 2019;2019:6214921.
8. Linet OI, Neff LL. Intracavernous prostaglandin E1 in erectile dysfunction. Clin Investig. 1994;72(2):139–49.
9. Zhao H, Berdahl C, Bresee C, Moradzadeh A, Houman J, Kim H, et al. Priapism from recreational intracavernosal injections in a high-risk metropolitan community. J Sex Med. 2019;16(10):1650–4.
10. Carneiro F, Nascimento B, Miranda EP, Cury J, Cerri GG, Chammas MC. Audiovisual sexual stimulation improves diagnostic accuracy of penile doppler ultrasound in patients with erectile dysfunction. J Sex Med. 2020;17(2):249–56.
11. Lowe FC, Jarow JP. Placebo-controlled study of oral terbutaline and pseudoephedrine in management of prostaglandin E1-induced prolonged erections. Urology. 1993;42(1):51–3; discussion 3–4.
12. Priyadarshi S. Oral terbutaline in the management of pharmacologically induced prolonged erection. Int J Impot Res. 2004;16(5):424–6.
13. Mishra K, Loeb A, Bukavina L, Baumgarten A, Beilan J, Mendez M, et al. Management of priapism: a contemporary review. Sex Med Rev. 2020;8(1):131–9.
14. Muneer A, Ralph D. Guideline of guidelines: priapism. BJU Int. 2017;119(2):204–8.
15. Okpala I, Westerdale N, Jegede T, Cheung B. Etilefrine for the prevention of priapism in adult sickle cell disease. Br J Haematol. 2002;118(3):918–21.
16. Gbadoé AD, Atakouma Y, Kusiaku K, Assimadi JK. Management of sickle cell priapism with etilefrine. Arch Dis Child. 2001;85(1):52–3.
17. Graham BA, Wael A, Jack C, Rohan MA, Wayne HJG. An overview of emergency pharmacotherapy for priapism. Expert Opin Pharmacother. 2022;23(12):1371–80.

Chapter 11
Evaluation of Penile Deformities in the Erect State of the Penis

11.1 Introduction

Peyronie's disease (PD) is a benign condition of the penis whose etiologic factors are still not fully understood. However, the most common suspected contributing factors encompass instances of sexual trauma in individuals with a genetic inclination toward abnormal wound healing, or as part of a broader context involving connective tissue disorders, autoimmune conditions, or arterial diseases. PD is characterized by the formation of fibrous tissue plaques within the tunica albuginea, usually causing a penile deformity.

While initially noted in 1561 by Fallopius and Vesalius, it was not until 1743 that Francois Gigot de la Peyronie provided a comprehensive description of the disease [1]. The real incidence of PD is still a matter of debate and may vary from 1 up to 16% [2]. However, many authors will agree that the real prevalence noted nowadays is considerably superior to what was previously suspected.

Congenital penile curvature (CPD) is another condition that leads to penile deformity that might require medical care [3]. This condition, often characterized by a noticeable bend in the erect state, with estimates suggesting it affects around 1–4% of the male population. While the exact cause remains multifactorial, factors such as genetic predisposition, fetal positioning, and variations in penile tissue development contribute to its occurrence. It usually affects a younger population that starts to note penile asymmetry during pubertal development [4].

Therefore, penile deformities can arise from various factors such as CPD, PD, and trauma, which might significantly impact both physical and psychological well-being of men. PDU emerges as a crucial diagnostic tool in comprehensively evaluating these deformities, providing insights into their etiology, severity, and implications for erectile function that will help guide treatment. Although it is a common practice to use autophotography to evaluate penile deformities and avoid

© The Author(s), under exclusive license to Springer Nature Switzerland AG 2024

E. d. P. Miranda, F. Carneiro, *Penile Color Duplex-Doppler Ultrasound in Erectile Dysfunction Diagnosis and Management*, https://doi.org/10.1007/978-3-031-55649-4_11

the hassles of in-office erection test coupled with PDU, it is the author's understanding that this strategy leads to an unreliable evaluation and should be therefore avoided [5].

11.2   Is It Worth Performing Ultrasound of the Flaccid Penis in Peyronie's Disease?

Overall, the diagnosis of PD is based on medical history and a clinical examination with plaque palpation. In theory, no further complementary test is required for establishing the diagnosis of PD in most cases. However, there are some instances in which performing US examination of the flaccid penis may be useful.

Ultrasound imaging of the flaccid penis in PD can provide essential etiological insights as it may capture structural anomalies such as plaques and fibrotic changes in cases where palpation is inconclusive or for atypical PD presentation [6]. Monitoring plaque changes is also a strategy used by some clinicians in order to discriminate between acute and chronic PD, though such findings may be eventually controversial.

Visualizing the extent of fibrotic changes might also aid in planning intralesional therapy, not to mention that these ultrasound findings enhance patient understanding and engagement. Finally, US images may be used as a medical document for insurance purposes to justify surgical or medical interventions.

However, it is the authors' suggestions that US in the flaccid state adds very little to the clinical decision-making process of penile deformities. In fact, a conventional PDU with an induced erection will serve for all these abovementioned functions and provide even more helpful information.

11.3   Plaque and Calcifications Measurements

Accurate assessment of penile deformities may involve meticulous measurements of plaques and calcifications [7]. With the use of high-resolution transducers, the most current US technology can accurately identify and measure calcified plaques. Thickening of the tunica albuginea without calcification can be also determined, and precise measurements of plaque dimensions may be performed. Though of limited utility, quantifying the length, width, and depth of plaques may offer objective data that might eventually guide treatment decisions and provide baseline information for monitoring progression. It has been used in clinical trials and is routinely used by many experts worldwide.

Calcifications within plaques are relatively easy to assess as they have remarkable hyperechoic images with posterior shadowing, as demonstrated in Fig. 11.1. Plaque calcification has been traditionally linked to stable PD or often associated with advanced PD. However, this concept has been recently questioned as many mild and acute PD may display a significant calcification burden.

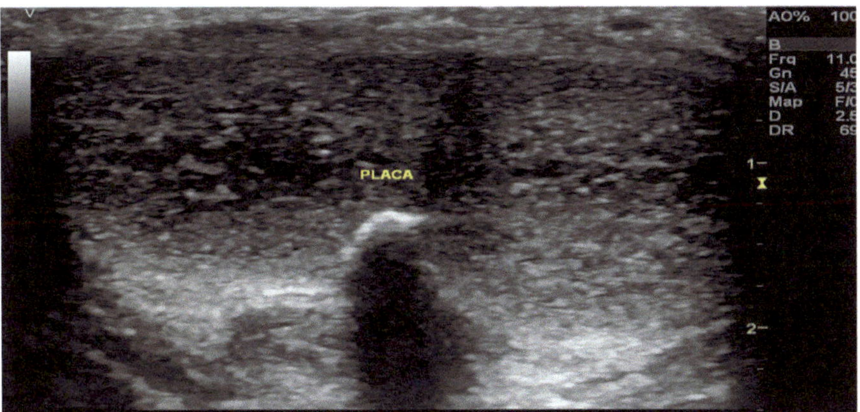

Fig. 11.1 B-Mode US demonstrating a calcified plaque with posterior shadowing

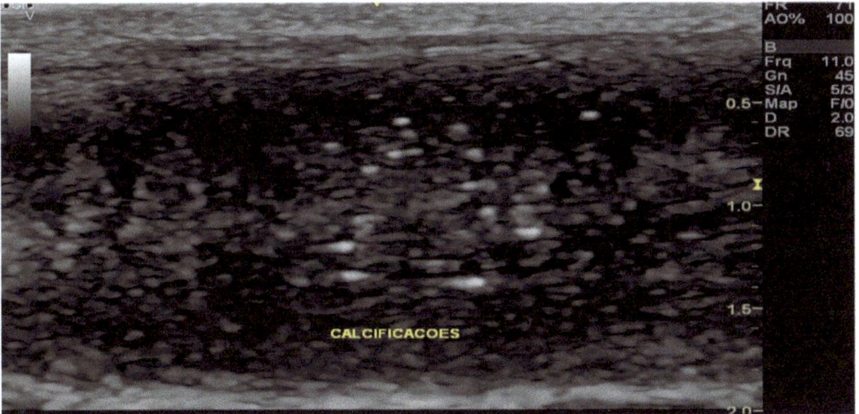

Fig. 11.2 Intracavernous calcification in a man with PD

The presence, location, and extent of calcifications offer clinicians information when considering treatments such as intralesional injections, which may require adjustments based on the extent of calcifications. Moreover, calcification might suggest a more intense inflammatory process that could eventually lead to surgical difficulties, particularly for grafting procedures or more complex penile reconstructive surgery.

The identification of intracavernosal calcifications is a different entity and is a common finding in men with PD [8]. Although it might not help in predicting deformity severity, they are usually associated with impaired erectile function as they suggest the presence of structural alterations in the cavernous tissue. Note that these calcifications as demonstrate in Fig. 11.2 are not exclusive for PD and might have an impact on erectile function in other clinical scenarios.

Some authors advocate that visualizing and measuring plaques and calcifications dynamically during the erect state might indicate disease severity and progression. Moreover, several studies have used these parameters as main treatment outcome measures [9]. However, the authors of the present book understand that although these findings may of importance in specific scenarios and might provide more information in PDU reports, they are not critical for the decision-making process and are therefore optional for those with more advanced US skills.

11.4   Evaluation of Erectile Function in the Curved Penis

Although the diagnosis of PD can be made solely on medical history and physical examination, the evaluation of ED in this patient population is far more problematic. It is a fact that ED questionnaires were not validated in men with PD and there might be significant confounding factors [10]. There is a high prevalence of ED in men with PD, and studies have suggested that many of these patients have psychogenic ED and tend eventually to underestimate their erectile function. If that is the case, many patients will have to undergo more invasive procedures as a result of a poor understanding of the exact magnitude of their erectile function.

In a study with 108 men with PD, 87 had diagnosis of ED according to validated questionnaires and of those 55% had normal vascular parameters, suggesting that there might be significant discordance between the IIEF and PDU [11]. Again, this overdiagnosis may exert considerable influence on treatment strategy, reinforcing the need of more specialized evaluation of erectile function in men with PD.

In this setting, PDU provides a dynamic assessment of erectile function through penile hemodynamic measure associated with rigidity and deformity assessment, including insights into how curvature influences erection biomechanics. By simultaneously evaluating penile curvature and hemodynamic changes, clinicians can correlate the anatomical deformity with functional alterations, helping to establish a comprehensive understanding of these issues.

11.5   Principles of Curvature Assessment

The most important principle in curvature assessment is that a rigid penis is required in order to perform an accurate procedure. Usually, the more rigid the penis, the more severe the deformity. Therefore, performing a curvature assessment with a suboptimal rigid may underestimate the deformity with potential severe consequences for treatment planning. That is also one of the reasons why autophotography is not ideal, as it is very difficult to assure adequate rigidity in these circumstances [5]. Compression on the base of the penis (basal compression) may temporarily increase intracavernosal pressure to allow for deformity assessment, but it is still not ideal. If for any reason the patient undergoing curvature assessment has significant

ED that is not responsive to ICI, then ED treatment with penile implant is usually mandatory [12].

11.5.1 Location, Direction, and Magnitude

Assessing penile curvature involves a comprehensive understanding of every aspect of the deformity and usually involves determination of location, direction, and magnitude. The idea is to provide an accurate documentation of every aspect of the curved penis to allow for an adequate treatment strategy.

First it is necessary to the indicate the curvature location or simple location along the shaft in which the deformity is found. Indicating the specific segment of the penis where the curvature occurs, whether proximal, midshaft, or distal, is recommended, although many variations of these denominations are possible. Then it is important to document the curvature's orientation, whether ventral, dorsal, lateral, biplanar, or complex. Understanding the direction informs clinicians about the nature of the deformity and guides decisions regarding diagnostic and therapeutic approaches.

Quantifying the magnitude of penile curvature is equally vital in assessing deformities. Using a goniometer (Fig. 11.3), it is possible to provide objective data on the exact degree of curvature. The precise measurement enhances diagnostic accuracy and influences treatment strategies, as PD severity is usually classified using 30° ranges: mild <30°, moderate between 30 and 60°, and severe >60°. Precise measurements of the curvature are perhaps the most important aspect of curvature assessment with an in-office erection test because it will influence treatment recommendations and outcomes entirely.

In summary, location, direction, and magnitude assessments enhance our ability to comprehensively understand and address deformities during the erect state and are crucial for surgical planning in cases of corrective procedures. These parameters aid in many aspects of the surgical procedure such as planning incisions, tissue manipulation, and postoperative expectations. Precise preoperative measurements contribute to surgical success and patient satisfaction. Examples of penile deformities during standard curvature assessments are shown in Figs. 11.4 and 11.5.

11.5.2 Assessment of Volume Loss

Evaluating the presence and extent of volume loss is a crucial dimension of penile curvature assessment and is commonly neglected [13].Volume loss often accompanies penile deformities, impacting both aesthetic appearance and functional aspects of the erect penis. During curvature assessments in PDU examinations, it is imperative to check for volume alterations, which is usually not a straightforward procedure. Most common deformities include indentation, tapering, and hourglass deformity, as illustrated in Fig. 11.6. Using flexible rulers, one can estimate volume

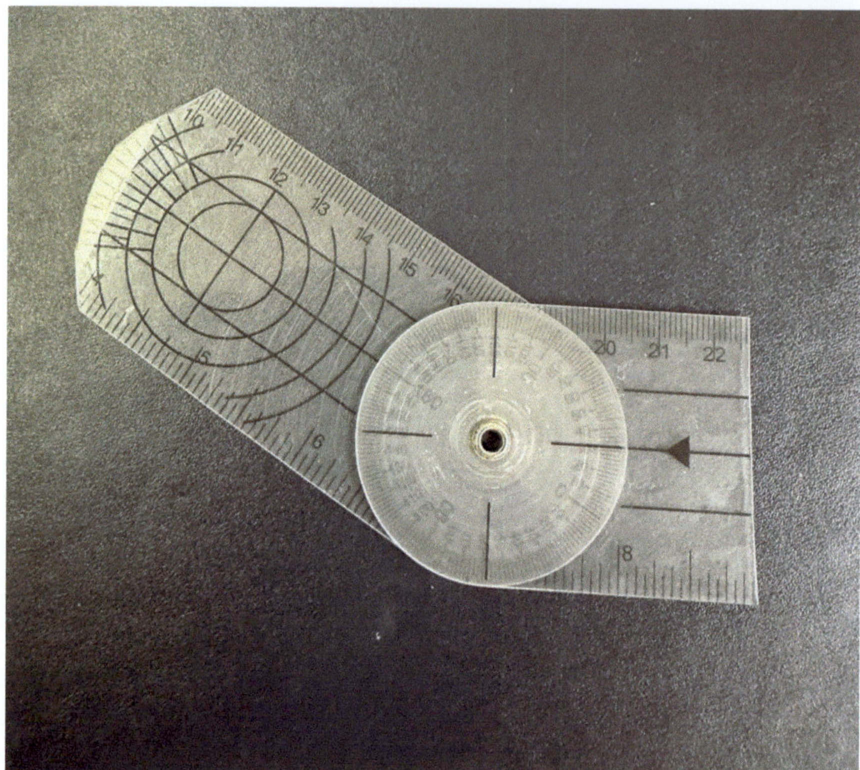

Fig. 11.3 Adapted goniometer ideal for curvature assessment

loss by comparing circumference difference between areas without significant narrowing and supposedly affected areas. However, sometimes deformities are complex, and these measures might not convey the detailed idea of the deformity. If that is the case, examiners should perform descriptive analysis of tunical defects or include pictures to register these nuances in order to provide insights into volume alterations, their impact on rigidity, aesthetics, and surgical treatments.

11.5.3   Assessment of Penile Instability

Penile instability is defined as the tendency of the penis to buckle during a rigid erection. It is commonly found in men with PD and consists of a significant problem for those individuals, as it contributes to difficulty with penetration and leads to increased patient bother and sexual dissatisfaction [14]. Penile instability is most likely in men with severe curvature and volume loss alteration such as hourglass deformity or indentation.

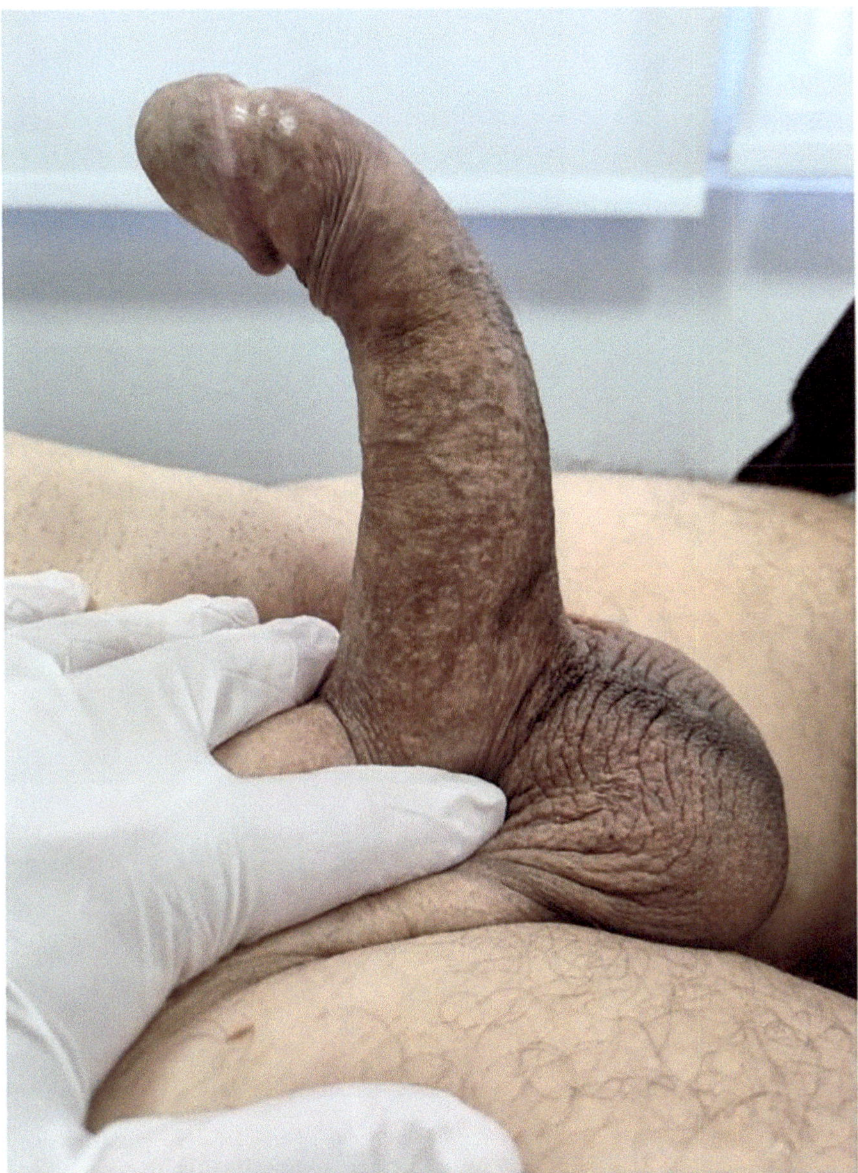

Fig. 11.4 Dorsal curvature of the penis

A precise measurement of the amount of axial load necessary to bend the penis would require a digital rigidometer, which is not universally available. Therefore, this measure may be performed in a more subjective manner by pressing against the glans penis, as demonstrated in Fig. 11.7a, b. The instability can also be classified as mild, moderate, or severe according to the examiner's subjective perspective.

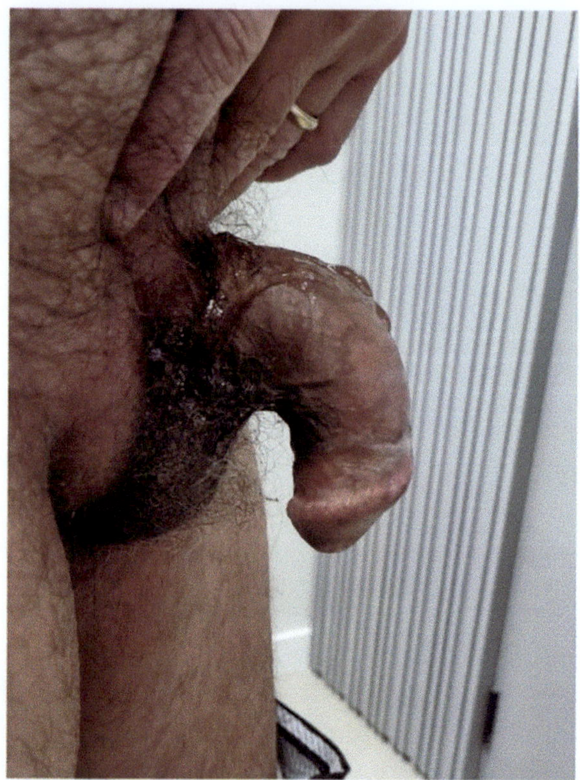

Fig. 11.5 Ventral curvature of the penis

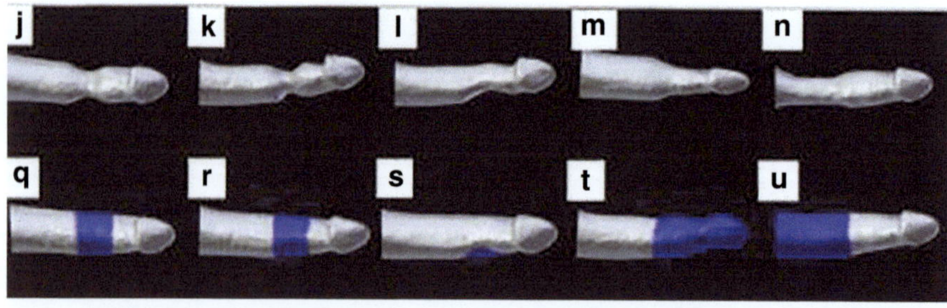

Fig. 11.6 Demonstration of common deformities with volume loss. J, K—hourglass deformity; L—indentation; M—distal tapering; N—proximal tapering. (Adapted from [13])

The assessment of penile instability guides treatment considerations for individuals with penile deformities. It may be helpful to understand penetration difficulties not related to ED. Severe instability as a result of the buckling effect is sometimes not corrected by simpler surgical procedures such as penile plication. Understanding how instability affects the deformity's behavior during erection informs decisions on interventions, including medical management, injections, or surgical correction.

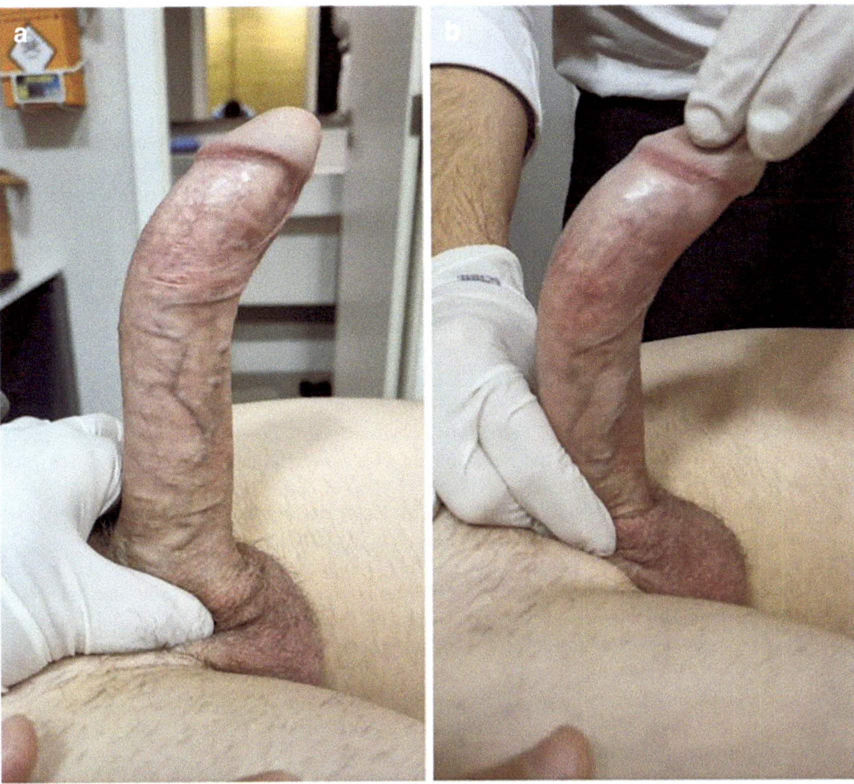

Fig. 11.7 (**a, b**) Demonstration of penile axial rigidity test by putting pressure against the glans penis during the erect state

11.6 Conclusions

The evaluation of penile deformities in the erect state with PDU adds depth to the understanding of these clinical entities and represents a fundamental step in the management of these conditions. This chapter has explored the multifaceted principles of PDU in men with penile deformities, most notably in PD, and the implications it holds for diagnosis, treatment, and patient-centered care. The combined evaluation of penile hemodynamics and detailed deformity assessment are critical for adequate care of patients with PD. By considering parameters such as location, direction, magnitude, volume alterations, and penile instability, clinicians gain a nuanced understanding of penile deformities that might optimize outcomes. Also, a more objective evaluation of erectile function is mandatory prior to corrective surgery. As clinicians become more familiar with its principles, applications, and interpretations, the integration of PDU into routine evaluations will undoubtedly improve the overall care and outcomes for individuals with penile deformities.

References

1. Musitelli S, Bossi M, Jallous H. A brief historical survey of "Peyronie's disease". J Sex Med. 2008;5(7):1737–46.
2. Al-Thakafi S, Al-Hathal N. Peyronie's disease: a literature review on epidemiology, genetics, pathophysiology, diagnosis and work-up. Transl Androl Urol. 2016;5(3):280–9.
3. Yachia D, Beyar M, Aridogan IA, Dascalu S. The incidence of congenital penile curvature. J Urol. 1993;150(5 Pt 1):1478–9.
4. Nyirády P, Kelemen Z, Bánfi G, Rusz A, Majoros A, Romics I. Management of congenital penile curvature. J Urol. 2008;179(4):1495–8.
5. Nascimento B, Cerqueira I, Miranda EP, Bessa J Jr, Ivanovic RF, Guglielmetti G, et al. Impact of camera deviation on penile curvature assessment using 2D pictures. J Sex Med. 2018;15(11):1638–44.
6. Liu Y, Zheng D, Liu X, Shi X, Shu S, Li J. Ultrasound on erect penis improves plaque identification in patients with Peyronie's disease. Front Pharmacol. 2019;10:312.
7. Levine L, Rybak J, Corder C, Farrel MR. Peyronie's disease plaque calcification—prevalence, time to identification, and development of a new grading classification. J Sex Med. 2013;10(12):3121–8.
8. Kalokairinou K, Konstantinidis C, Domazou M, Kalogeropoulos T, Kosmidis P, Gekas A. US imaging in Peyronie's disease. J Clin Imaging Sci. 2012;2:63.
9. Chung E, Yan H, De Young L, Brock GB. Penile Doppler sonographic and clinical characteristics in Peyronie's disease and/or erectile dysfunction: an analysis of 1500 men with male sexual dysfunction. BJU Int. 2012;110(8):1201–5.
10. Patel P, Masterson T, Ramasamy R. Penile duplex: clinical indications and application. Int J Impot Res. 2019;31(4):298–9.
11. Masterson TA 3rd, Efimenko IV, Nackeeran S, Parmar M, Ramasamy R. Discordant erectile function assessment between validated questionnaire scores and penile Doppler ultrasound in Peyronie's disease. Int J Impot Res. 2022;34(5):452–5.
12. Nehra A, Alterowitz R, Culkin DJ, Faraday MM, Hakim LS, Heidelbaugh JJ, et al. Peyronie's disease: AUA guideline. J Urol. 2015;194(3):745–53.
13. Margolin EJ, Mlynarczyk CM, Mulhall JP, Stember DS, Stahl PJ. Three-dimensional photography for quantitative assessment of penile volume-loss deformities in Peyronie's disease. J Sex Med. 2017;14(6):829–33.
14. Al Ansari A, Talib RA, Canguven O, Shamsodini A. Axial penile rigidity influences patient and partner satisfaction after penile prosthesis implantation. Arch Ital Urol Androl. 2013;85(3):138–42.

Chapter 12
Interpretation and Clinical Implications of Penile Hemodynamic Parameters

12.1 Introduction

The assessment of penile hemodynamic parameters through Doppler ultrasound has revolutionized our understanding of erectile function and vascular health.

The dynamic interplay between blood flow and penile tissues is central to achieving and maintaining a proper erection. Hemodynamic parameters, such as peak systolic velocity (PSV), end-diastolic velocity (EDV), resistive index (RI), and pulsatility index (PI), offer insights into the vascular health of the penile arteries [1]. By quantifying blood flow velocities and indices, clinicians can differentiate between normal hemodynamics, arterial insufficiency, and cavernous veno-occlusive dysfunction (CVOD). The correct interpretation of these penile hemodynamic parameters may guide therapeutic decisions in the management of ED. Understanding the specific vascular issues affecting erectile function informs the selection of appropriate interventions, such as oral medications, injection therapies, vacuum devices, or surgical procedures [2]. This individualized approach improves treatment efficacy and patient satisfaction.

12.2 Normative Parameters

Normative parameters serve as reference values that aid in discerning deviations from the typical vascular profile. These baseline values, often determined from healthy individuals without ED, provide a benchmark against which hemodynamic measurements are compared. Clinicians use these benchmarks to evaluate the significance of abnormalities in blood flow velocities and indices.

Key penile hemodynamic parameters commonly evaluated include peak systolic velocity (PSV), end-diastolic velocity (EDV), resistive index (RI), and pulsatility index (PI) measured in the main cavernosal artery. These measurements reflect the blood flow characteristics within the penile arteries during different phases of the cardiac cycle. There are also other possible parameters such as acceleration time (AT) in the cavernous arteries or even velocities in the profound dorsal vein, which have been described in the literature. However, it is the authors' understanding that evaluating multiple variables will not necessarily increase PDU's accuracy and will eventually make results more confusing and the examination more time consuming. To standardize and simplify PDU interpretation, the authors suggest utilizing PSVs and EDVs alone for the purpose of understanding penile hemodynamics. Even RIs, which have been extensively described in the literature and are considered one of the most traditional parameters to diagnose and classify CVOD, may have considerable variations, especially in case with very high PSVs.

12.2.1 Suggested Cutoffs

PDU provides peak systolic velocity (PSV) and end-diastolic velocity (EDV) to diagnose arterial insufficiency as well as veno-occlusive dysfunction. Several different values have been reported in the literature. Different cutoff points will yield different sensitivity and specificity values, with implications on diagnostic accuracy.

In general, the accepted thresholds for normal systolic and diastolic blood flow velocities in relation to the cavernosal arteries, subsequent to the injection of intra-cavernosal vasoactive agents, are commonly considered to be a peak systolic velocity (PSV) ranging from 25 to 35 cm/s and an end-diastolic velocity (EDV) lower than 3–5 cm/s [3].

While the American Urological Association (AUA) ED Guidelines suggest that PSVs<30 cm/s is considered evidence of arterial insufficiency and EDV> 5 cm/s is consistent with veno-occlusive dysfunction [2], the European Association of Urology (EAU) Guidelines suggest a lower EDV cutoff of>3 cm/s to be considered abnormal [4]. The normative criteria suggested by the authors are demonstrated in Table 12.1, which are in accordance with AUA guidelines.

Although there are some published criteria for defining mixed etiology for ED, which means the presence of arterial insufficiency and CVOD combined, we believe that PDU has not enough accuracy for such diagnosis. As the diagnosis of CVOD required a PSV >30 cm/s, those below that range will be classified as arterial

Table 12.1 Normative criteria for PDU

Final diagnosis	PSV	EDV
Normal hemodynamics	≥30 cm/s	<5 cm/s
Arterial insufficiency	<30 cm/s	<5 cm/s
CVOD	≥30 cm/s	≥5 cm/s

insufficiency. Therefore, in order to provide a precise diagnosis of mixed penile vascular dysfunction in men with PSV <30 cm, cavernosometry test is required. Nevertheless, classifying an eventual patient with an abnormal PDU study as arterial insufficiency instead of mixed dysfunction will represent no harm in terms of counseling and prognosis.

Another common confounding situation during PDU is the presence of unilateral dysfunction, when an asymmetric range of hemodynamic parameters is found between right and left cavernosal arteries. It has been suggested that lateral differences of PSV >10 cm/s represent a sign of unilateral arterial insufficiency [5]. However, the authors do not recommend using relative right-left asymmetries in PSV values to define unilateral arterial insufficiency as many factors may contribute to this finding. Instead, low absolute values should be preferably used (unilateral PSV <30 cm/s).

On the other hand, the diagnosis of unilateral CVOD is theoretically not adequate, since the cavernosal bodies represent a unique chamber of resistance. Though these differences do exist and may be commonly found, in the authors' experience the most common reason for unilateral arterial insufficiency or asymmetric EDVs is loss of erection during the examination, device maladjustments (angle, gain, scale, etc.), or even anatomic variations (multiple cavernosal arteries).

12.2.2   Hemodynamic Parameters in the Flaccid State of the Penis

It is the authors' current understanding the hemodynamic parameters in flaccid state do not necessarily reflect the vascular status in the erect state of the penis. Although it has been suggested that PSV >13 cm/s is highly predictive of cardiovascular disease [6], in clinical practice it was not demonstrated to be able to predict arterial insufficiency in the erect state [7]. In fact, the changes in vascular bed of cavernosal arteries and in the erectile tissue after ICI injection are usually not predictable. Therefore, routine evaluation of Doppler parameters in the flaccid state does not add diagnostic value to PDU, though they may be eventually performed according to examiner's preference or specific situations.

12.3   Normal PDU Indicates No Erectile Dysfunction?

ED is a multifactorial condition influenced by physiological, psychological, and vascular factors. While PDU provides valuable insights into penile hemodynamics, ED diagnosis encompasses a broader scope of factors, including psychological aspects, relationship dynamics, and patient-reported experiences. Therefore, PDU does not rule out the diagnosis ED, as clinical aspects are determinants for this diagnosis [8, 9].

A normal PDU reflects healthy hemodynamic parameters during sexual stimulation, indicating efficient arterial inflow and venous outflow. This piece of information is relevant for clinicians and patients and may serve as an important milestone in their ED journey. In that scenario, psychological factors, hormonal imbalances, and neurological issues can contribute to ED despite normal hemodynamic parameters and should be extensively investigated [10]. Also, patients with normal PDU might have signs of endothelial dysfunction or initial vascular dysfunctions that are compensated by intracavernosal vasoactive agents that induce complete smooth muscle relaxation [11]. In these cases, although the exact diagnosis remains still unknown, the fact that they are responsive to pharmacotherapy holds significant prognostic implications and aids in therapy adjustments.

Understanding that a normal PDU does not definitively indicate the absence of ED is crucial for clinical practice. Clinicians should interpret PDU findings within the broader context of patient history and reported symptoms. ED diagnosis involves a multifaceted evaluation that considers psychological, physiological, and vascular factors. Integrating patient-reported symptoms, psychological factors, medical history, and PDU results leads to a comprehensive diagnosis that guides personalized treatment strategies.

12.4   Implications of Normal PDU Studies

A normal penile Doppler ultrasound (PDU) study carries significant implications for clinical practice, patient counseling, and treatment decisions.

First, a normal PDU study provides reassurance regarding the patient's penile vascular health. Clinicians can use these findings to alleviate patient concerns and focus on addressing potential non-vascular factors contributing to erectile dysfunction. This is particularly useful for a significant number of reluctant patients with psychogenic ED, in which normal PDU results can prompt further exploration of psychological factors contributing to ED. By ruling out significant vascular issues, clinicians can delve more deeply into the psychological dimensions of the condition. Open communication with patients about stress, anxiety, and performance-related concerns allows for comprehensive treatment planning.

For individuals with normal PDU studies, treatment strategies can be tailored to target specific contributing factors. Normal PDU results prompt discussions about lifestyle and behavioral modifications. Clinicians can collaborate with patients to implement healthier habits, such as weight management, exercise, and stress reduction. These changes support overall vascular health and contribute to improved erectile function.

Also, in cases where ICI is deemed appropriate, PDU studies may serve as a starting point for optimal medication selection and dose titration [12].

Educating patients about the significance of normal PDU findings fosters better understanding of their condition. Patients can grasp the interplay between vascular health, psychological factors, and erectile function. This knowledge empowers individuals to actively participate in their treatment journey.

In summary, for patients with normal PDU studies and ED, the possible etiologic factors include psychogenic ED, neurogenic ED, biomechanical problems (such as found in penile deformities), or endothelial dysfunction. Understanding the implications of normal PDU studies is of paramount importance for those who perform it, especially because in the setting that an adequate PDU technique with redosing strategies are utilized, the majority of PDU exams tend to be normal. That happens because of the high efficacy of ICI to promote smooth muscle relaxation and compensate minor vascular issues. Therefore, PDU examiners must learn how to translate this information in the patient's benefit.

12.5   Implications of Abnormal PDU Studies

On the other hand, abnormal findings in properly conducted PDU studies indicate a permanent damage to the penile vascular physiology that will eventually require more invasive therapies if penetrative intercourse is desired. It carries significant clinical implications, as it demonstrates a compromised blood flow reflecting the extent of vascular or erectile tissue damage.

Most patients in this scenario will be good candidates for penile implant surgery. Although high-dose ICI alone or in combination with other strategies may be also offered, it usually leads to more inconsistent results in terms of penetration ability and satisfaction rates [13, 14].

Here is the importance of ethics during PDU conduction. As PDU is highly operator-dependent, abnormal results may be deliberately achieved with poor-quality exams to suggest the undue need of more invasive therapies and promote financial profit. Unfortunately, this practice is still very common worldwide and has to certain point undermine PDU credibility over the years. We strongly advocate that these practices be avoided at all costs, and the patients' wellbeing be the primary goal of every ED clinic and PDU examiner.

12.6   Further Interpretation of Penile Hemodynamic Studies

Interpreting PDU studies involves more than direct measurements of Doppler parameters. It is a comprehensive hemodynamic test, that usually requires a thorough understanding of penile physiology and continuous monitoring of the different stages of an erection. Moreover, PDU consists of direct evaluation of ICI response. Instead of focusing solely on the final diagnosis of PDU, or even in the dichotomy normal vs. abnormal findings, it is important to observe the whole context in which the exam was performed. This includes amount of ICI required to achieve a given erection status with specific hemodynamic parameters and the eventual need of erection reversal at the end of the examination. Analyzing these factors altogether may shed light on difficult or inconclusive diagnosis and may guide clinicians to translate the obtained information into clinical practice.

12.7   Prognostic Value of PDU

PDU studies carry implications for long-term erectile function and offer valuable prognostic insights that guide treatment decisions and provide a glimpse into the potential outcomes of therapeutic interventions.

In fact, the real utility of PDU in predicting prognostic value has been questioned in the literature [15–17]. In the series published by Morgado et al., PDU has not demonstrated to be superior to IIEF alone. However, in these studies, the authors compared hemodynamic parameters to IIEF in a continuous fashion, which is not the purpose of PDU. In other words, patients with PSV >80 cm/s do not have better prognosis than those with PSV >60 cm/s. There are other nuances that are usually neglected and might have relevant prognostic value such as ICI dosing during PDU within the same diagnostic spectrum. Patients reaching normal hemodynamic parameters with high dose of ICI (>50 UI or 0.5 mL) usually have different outcomes than those needing only low doses or even requiring reversal. The same concept is eventually applicable for those with compensated arterial insufficiency. For example, a 50-year-old patient that required 40 units of trimix to achieve a 8/10 rigidity and displayed atherosclerotic disease in the left cavernosal artery with a PSV of 24 cm/s would most likely behave differently in the long term if after 5 units of trimix the same patient had 10/10 rigidity and PSV of 57 cm/s with need of reversal agents in the end. In the first scenario, the patient had a compensated arterial insufficiency, while the second represents a completely normal hemodynamic with an intact vascular anatomy. These nuances would never be noticed with IIEF and ICI test alone, highlighting the potential impact of PDU on ED prognosis.

12.8   PDU Results and Clinical Decision-Making in Erectile Dysfunction

PDU results play a pivotal role in shaping clinical decision-making for individuals with ED. As previously discussed in this chapter, there are several clinical implications according to PDU findings. Whether pharmacological, psychological, or surgical interventions are considered, PDU findings provide clinicians with an objective assessment of penile hemodynamics, guiding the selection of interventions that align with the underlying vascular issues.

Patients with normal PDU studies usually have more treatment options available, while those with abnormal findings will eventually require more invasive therapies.

For individuals seeking non-invasive or conservative interventions, PDU results offer insights into the efficacy of treatments like phosphodiesterase type 5 inhibitors (PDE5i), ICI, and eventually low-intensity shock wave therapy [2, 4]. Those with severe vascular dysfunction are candidates more suitable for high doses of concentrated ICI therapies or penile implants.

It is important to mention that PDU does not provide specific indication for any type of treatment modality. Instead, shared decision-making between clinicians and patients thrives on the transparency provided by PDU results. Patients actively participate in treatment discussions, understanding the correlation between PDU findings, treatment options, and expected outcomes. For example, a 61-year-old patient with normal hemodynamics with a high dose of ICI might choose to proceed with a penile implant though being a good candidate for ICI therapy, if proper counseling is given.

12.9   Conclusions

The interpretation and clinical implications of penile hemodynamic parameters through PDU studies represent a cornerstone in the comprehensive understanding and management of ED. Through normative parameters and dynamic interpretation, clinicians gain insights into the intricate interplay of arterial inflow and tissue resistance, contributing to a more robust understanding of penile vascular health. The significance of both normal and abnormal PDU studies extends beyond the realm of hemodynamics, encompassing psychosocial, psychological, and lifestyle factors that contribute to erectile function.

As a diagnostic tool, PDU studies provide a window into the diverse etiologies of ED, allowing clinicians to tailor interventions based on the specific vascular challenges present. The prognostic value of PDU findings guides treatment expectations and allows for informed treatment selection and shared decision-making, empowering patients to actively engage in their healthcare journey. In conclusion, dynamic interpretation of penile hemodynamic studies is essential for a nuanced understanding of ED.

References

1. Carneiro F, Saito OC, Miranda EP. Standardization of penile hemodynamic evaluation through color duplex-Doppler ultrasound. Rev Assoc Med Bras (1992). 2020;66(9):1180–6.
2. Burnett AL, Nehra A, Breau RH, Culkin DJ, Faraday MM, Hakim LS, et al. Erectile dysfunction: AUA guideline. J Urol. 2018;200(3):633–41.
3. Cavallini G, Scroppo FI, Zucchi A. Peak systolic velocity thresholds of cavernosal penile arteries in patients with and without risk factors for arterial erectile deficiency. Andrology. 2016;4(6):1187–92.

4. Salonia A, Bettocchi C, Boeri L, Capogrosso P, Carvalho J, Cilesiz NC, et al. European Association of Urology guidelines on sexual and reproductive health-2021 update: male sexual dysfunction. Eur Urol. 2021;80(3):333–57.

5. Varela CG, Yeguas LAM, Rodríguez IC, Vila MDD. Penile Doppler ultrasound for erectile dysfunction: technique and interpretation. AJR Am J Roentgenol. 2020;214(5):1112–21.

6. Corona G, Fagioli G, Mannucci E, Romeo A, Rossi M, Lotti F, et al. Penile doppler ultrasound in patients with erectile dysfunction (ED): role of peak systolic velocity measured in the flaccid state in predicting arteriogenic ED and silent coronary artery disease. J Sex Med. 2008;5(11):2623–34.

7. Cannarella R, Calogero AE, Aversa A, Condorelli RA, La Vignera S. Differences in penile hemodynamic profiles in patients with erectile dysfunction and anxiety. J Clin Med. 2021;10(3):402.

8. Butaney M, Thirumavalavan N, Hockenberry MS, Kirby EW, Pastuszak AW, Lipshultz LI. Variability in penile duplex ultrasound international practice patterns, technique, and interpretation: an anonymous survey of ISSM members. Int J Impot Res. 2018;30(5):237–42.

9. Cormio L, Nisén H, Selvaggi FP, Ruutu M. A positive pharmacological erection test does not rule out arteriogenic erectile dysfunction. J Urol. 1996;156(5):1628–30.

10. Nascimento B, Miranda EP, Terrier JE, Carneiro F, Mulhall JP. A critical analysis of methodology pitfalls in duplex Doppler ultrasound in the evaluation of patients with erectile dysfunction: technical and interpretation deficiencies. J Sex Med. 2020;17(8):1416–22.

11. Aversa A, Bruzziches R, Francomano D, Natali M, Gareri P, Spera G. Endothelial dysfunction and erectile dysfunction in the aging man. Int J Urol. 2010;17(1):38–47.

12. Aversa A, Crafa A, Greco EA, Chiefari E, Brunetti A, La Vignera S. The penile duplex ultrasound: how and when to perform it? Andrology. 2021;9(5):1457–66.

13. Chen J, Godschalk MF, Katz PG, Mulligan T. Combining intracavernous injection and external vacuum as treatment for erectile dysfunction. J Urol. 1995;153(5):1476–7.

14. Cai Z, Song X, Zhang J, Yang B, Li H. Practical approaches to treat ED in PDE5i nonresponders. Aging Dis. 2020;11(5):1202–18.

15. Morgado A, Dinis P, Silva CM. Is there a role for bilateral peak systolic velocity readings in a penile duplex ultrasound? Andrologia. 2019;51(8):e13297.

16. Morgado A, Diniz P, Silva CM. Is there a point to performing a penile duplex ultrasound? J Sex Med. 2019;16(10):1574–80.

17. Silva AC, Silva CM, Morgado A. Erection hardness score or penile Doppler ultrasound: which is a better predictor of failure of nonsurgical treatment of erectile dysfunction? Sex Med. 2023;11(2):qfad009.

Chapter 13
Step-by-Step Guide for Penile Doppler Ultrasound Examinations: Practical Tips

13.1   Introduction

In 1985, Lue et al. introduced the procedure of penile duplex Doppler ultrasound (PDU) as an alternative to evaluating blood flow during an erection [1]. At that time, PDU was considered a less invasive methodology of erectile hemodynamics evaluation in comparison to dynamic infusion cavernosometry and cavernosography and selective internal pudendal arteriography.

Peak systolic velocity (PSV), which gives direct assessment of the arterial supply, end-diastolic velocity (EDV), and resistive index (RI), which indirectly evaluates the veno-occlusive mechanism, is the standard hemodynamic parameters examined [2]. Despite decades of experience since it was first described, and several efforts to standardize the procedure, there is still considerable heterogeneity in published PDU protocols, including different intracavernosal vasoactive agents, variability in redosing schedules, different methods for assessing erectile rigidity, timing of hemodynamic assessment, and different hemodynamic parameter cutoffs [3].

The lack of standardized hemodynamic evaluation through PDU is one of the main limitations of this method [4]. It explains the wide variation in conducting and interpreting penile hemodynamic tests in clinical practice and scientific research. These characteristics have contributed to the widespread perception that PDU is untrustworthy, as it can lead to erroneous treatment protocols [5].

The purpose of this chapter is to provide standard operating techniques to minimize confounders in order to predict the etiology of ED in an accurate manner. This is a step-by-step guide with some practical suggestions for making PDU more reliable and reproducible.

E. d. P. Miranda, F. Carneiro, *Penile Color Duplex-Doppler Ultrasound in Erectile Dysfunction Diagnosis and Management*,
https://doi.org/10.1007/978-3-031-55649-4_13

13.2 Exam Preparation

PDU can be performed in either outpatient clinics or hospitals, as long as these locations are adequately equipped. Vascular ultrasonography of the penis is dynamic and requires one or more intracavernous injection (ICI) of vasodilating drugs to assist the patient in achieving a rigid erection. In order to execute an accurate interpretation, examiners must be knowledgeable with the physiology of erection and be able to identify numerous confounding factors and artifacts. In addition, the examiner must be able to diagnose and/or treat ICI-related prolonged erections and priapism.

13.3 Technical Prep Work

A. About the Location

- PDU must be performed in a quiet location due to the influence of psychological and environmental factors on the erectile response.
- Equipment to provide audio-visual sexual stimuli is an interesting tool because it helps patients to get a more rigid erection with lower doses of vasoactive agents. It is important to be conscious about the diverse sexual orientation and preference of each individual, so ideally the patient should be able to choose among different options available.
- Medication vials must be properly stored; these include vasoactive agents and sympathomimetics for erection reversal. Vasoactive agents with alprostadil must be stored in a refrigerator as it is thermolabile.

B. About the Ultrasound Device

- Ultrasound instrument with Doppler
- High-frequency linear transducer (7.5–18 MHz)
- Imaging storage device and printer

13.4 Exam Conduction

The penis is initially in a flaccid state during the PDU exam. A high-frequency linear transducer (7.5–18 MHz) must be used to scan the entire penis in mode B using longitudinal and cross-sectional pictures. This initial evaluation provides an overview of potential major alterations in the tunica albuginea and the erectile tissue's ecotexture. This scanning is ideally performed in the ventral aspect of the penis, with the patient holding the glans towards the umbilical scar.

At the start of the examination, measurements of the internal diameter of the cavernous arteries (right and left) as well as, optionally, the peak systolic velocity (PSV) in the cavernous arteries in spectral Doppler mode can be made. Although some studies have shown promising predictive PSV values in a flaccid state, the general agreement is that PDU should be performed with a drug-induced erection [2, 6, 7]. In other words, vasoactive drugs must be always used in order to obtain reliable hemodynamic parameters, as PDU in the flaccid state adds very little to the diagnostic accuracy of this method [8–10].

Although there is no consensus on the ideal drug combination or dose to be used for inducing an erection, it is anticipated that the dose will be the lowest necessary to produce a rigid erection (EHS 4). If obtaining such rigidity is not possible, at the very least the best quality erection (BQE) in other circumstances should be achieved, which commonly required redosing of ICI. Since every patient responds differently to intracavernous medication, there is no pre-established efficacious dosage that can be utilized universally. A redosing approach based on periodic reassessments of penile rigidity can counterbalance the adrenergic effect and enable adequate smooth muscle relaxation. Again, the ideal drug or combination, dose, and number of injections during redosing protocols are still a matter of debate [11]. We recommend starting with 0.05–0.1 mL of trimix combination of papaverine 30 mg/mL, phentolamine 1 mg/mL, and alprostadil 10 mcg/mL.

Practical tip #1: Inquiring about previous ICI use and clinical response as well as comorbidities and severity of ED is usually helpful in determining the initial dose. The presence of rigid nocturnal erections is another important predictor for determining lower initial ICI dose.

Practical tip #2: We recommend using a rigidity-based redosing protocol with no more than three doses. The subsequent dose is defined according to penile rigidity. We believe more than three doses is not necessary and is excessively time-consuming. If BQE is not reached after three doses, consider repeating the process later, if applicable.

The transducer should be positioned at the base of the penis in the penoscrotal junction during cavernous artery assessment. The cavernous arteries might theoretically be evaluated at any point along their extent since cavernous bodies are tridimensional structures that function as a single chamber. However, several research have already examined the impact of transducer position, and they have demonstrated that proximal assessments could overestimate PSV values while distal evaluations might underestimate EDVs [12]. To prevent artifacts brought on by excessively proximal or too distal placements, we generally advise taking the readings on the ventral face, near the penoscrotal junction.

Practical tip #3: Placing the probe under the testicles is sometimes a helpful way to reach cavernous arteries in an advantageous position for scanning proximally. In a longitudinal plane, the arteries will be verticalized and have a decent length and favorable Doppler angle. Remember to avoid excessive pressure on the crura to avoid vessel closure.

13.5   Step-by-Step Guide for PDU Examination

- To begin the examination, turn on the ultrasound machine and choose the suitable setups for the transducer.
- Describe to the patient every step of the evaluation process and obtain his permission to continue.
- Instruct the patient to relax as much as possible while in dorsally decubitus (laying flat).
- To begin scanning, place the transducer with transmitter gel on the base of the penis (penoscrotal junction).
- Examine the corpus cavernousum and spongiosum's anatomical structures and note any abnormalities in the ecotexture. Always scan and photograph your documentation in both transverse and longitudinal planes.
- Register images of the two cavernous arteries in cross-section and longitudinally (at the proximal third of the penile shaft) and note any potential anatomical differences. The left and right cavernous arteries' intraluminal diameters should be measured, together with the proper nomenclature.
- To measure the PSV [13], activate the Doppler mode and adjust the sample and angle (to a maximum of 60°). Apply the same technique to each cavernous artery and mark the laterality in the records.
- Hold the penis firmly while injecting the vasodilator into the center or proximal third of the penile shaft, away from the dorsal neural bundle, using a syringe (0.5–3 mL) and insulin needle (27–30 gauge, 0.5 in). For 10 s, press the injection site to prevent reflux of the medication into superficial planes. Record the time the medication was administered for a tighter time monitoring.
- While watching an erotic film, encourage patients to engage in self-stimulation.

> ***Practical tip 4:*** *ICI of vasoactive drugs can be eventually challenging. The patient's anatomic characteristics may be unfavorable. For example in cases of buried penis, Peyronie's disease, or if the patient has very high levels of adrenaline at the time of injection, which may contribute to excessive contraction of the penis, there may be doubt on whether the drug was delivered to the correct location. In such cases, injecting a small quantity of air together with the medication within the syringe might be helpful, because the gas causes a sound reverberation artifact and generates a hyperechogenic image, so you can be certain that you have injected the medication into the cavernous body.*

To do this, the patient must be alone in the examination room for an adequate amount of time to develop smooth muscle relaxation. Ten minutes of manual and audiovisual stimulation tend to be enough for the first scanning evaluation [4, 14].

– PSV and EDV are the most important hemodynamic Doppler parameters, and they must be assessed at the peak of the erection. Seriated measurements and seriated rigidity assessment are essential for evaluating the dynamic process of erection. However, it is very important that the primary measurement be obtained and recorded at the highest rigidity (EHS 4 or BQE).
– Measure the intraluminal diameter on both sides while taking cross-sectional and longitudinal pictures of the cavernous arteries at the BQE or EHS 4. Record the data that was acquired and the appropriate laterality.
– Ask the patient to wait between 30 min and 1 h following the assessment so you can check for any potential adverse effects, such as prolonged erection, priapism, or pain /discomfort in penis.
– Reversing the patient's prolonged painful erection is worthwhile in order to prevent priapism. Since persistent erections lasting longer than 1 h might result in cavernous body edema, which significantly diminishes the patient's sensitivity to sympathomimetic drugs and increases the likelihood of eventual aspiration, we do not advise waiting up to 4 h to do proceed with reversal protocols. For detumescence, it is possible to administer an alpha-adrenergic selective agonist (such as 200–300 mcg of phenylephrine or 5–10 mg of etilefrine, as discussed in Chap. 10) into the cavernous body every 10 min up to three injections. Although countless injections are plausible, we believe that they become time-consuming and deteriorate the patient's experience, similarly to the erection-induction protocol. Having a pre-established protocol with a maximum number of injections is interesting for both patient and provider. A cardiac monitor must be used to keep track of symptoms including acute hypertension, headaches, reflex bradycardia, tachycardia, palpitations, or cardiac arrhythmias. Serial blood pressure readings must also be collected. If detumescence does not occur, the patient must undergo cavernous body aspiration for a prompt resolution.
– The examination report must be thorough and include at least the concentrations and the amount of medication given, the maximum rigidity obtained, PSV and EDV in the peak rigidity, and the necessity of erection reversal. We also recommend that the report should include clinical impressions such as patient anxiety throughout the exam, among other subjective perceptions.
– Schedule a follow-up appointment whenever necessary, discharge the patient, and provide him with general orientations and cautions such as how to proceed in case of late onset of priapism.
– Include the report and any authorized photographs in the patient's medical file.

13.6 Recording Relevant Findings

The proper recording of data is essential since it shows that patients are receiving high-quality care. The exam date, patient name, and anatomical structure names must all be included in the images. For clinical and legal reasons, it is essential to maintain permanent records of all examinations and medical reports. Additionally, it is crucial to provide a detailed explanation of the following factors:

1. It is critical to document the patient's pertinent data, such as age, dosage, and medicine type. Ideally, the following evaluated parameters should be recorded:

    (a) PSV, EDV, and eventually RI at maximum rigidity during the two cavernous arteries' investigation
    (b) The total amount of medication administered, which should be the sum of all injections performed during the examination
    (c) Similarly, the total amount of sympathomimetic administered in the detumescence phase of PDU, if required
    (d) The left and right cavernous arteries' longitudinal and cross-sectional widths both before and after pharmacological induction (optional)

2. Data evaluation and interpretation

    (a) Rigidity information throughout PDU hemodynamic assessment of the penis must also be recorded, ideally using the EHS or the decimal erection scale.
    (b) It is important to note structural anomalies in the arteries and the penis related to the tunica albuginea, corpus cavernous, and spongy (heterogeneity, hyperechoic regions, and plaques).
    (c) It is important to identify Doppler artifacts like aliasing, acoustic shadowing, and mirror images, among others [15].
    (d) At specific sections of the cavernosal vascular branches, primarily in bifurcations, ramifications, stenoses, and regions distal to plaques, it might be challenging to correctly interpret the direction of blood flow. The positioning of the transducer and how the angle is used are just two of the factors that affect variations in blood flow direction. To prevent inaccurate assessments and interpretations, the examiner must be able to perform fine adjustments in the US device [16].

13.7 Conclusion

Evaluation of penile hemodynamics using PDU through a standard approach requires training. This chapter has summarized a step-by-step approach with practical tips that may be helpful for beginners. Although each examiners will eventually develop one's own preferences, the most important pillars that should never be forgotten are the utilization redosing strategies during erection induction, the use of a rigidity-based evaluation protocol of hemodynamic parameters, and to always be conscious about the need of an effective detumescence protocol using reversal agents.

References

1. Lue T, Mueller S, Jow Y, Hwang T. Functional evaluation of penile arteries with duplex ultrasound in vasodilator-induced erection. Urol Clin North Am. 1989;16(4):799–807.
2. Aversa A, Sarteschi LM. The role of penile color-duplex ultrasound for the evaluation of erectile dysfunction. J Sex Med. 2007;4(5):1437–47.
3. Nascimento B, Miranda EP, Terrier J-E, Carneiro F, Mulhall JP. A critical analysis of methodology pitfalls in duplex Doppler ultrasound in the evaluation of patients with erectile dysfunction: technical and interpretation deficiencies. J Sex Med. 2020;17(8):1416–22.
4. Lee B, Sikka SC, Randrup ER, Villemarette P, Baum N, Hower JF, et al. Standardization of penile blood flow parameters in normal men using intracavernous prostaglandin E1 and visual sexual stimulation. J Urol. 1993;149(1):49–52.
5. Cavallini G, Maretti C. Unreliability of the duplex scan in diagnosing corporeal venous occlusive disease in young healthy men with erectile deficiency. Urology. 2018;113:91–8.
6. Hsiao W, Shrewsberry AB, Moses KA, Pham D, Ritenour CW. Longer time to peak flow predicts better arterial flow parameters on penile Doppler ultrasound. Urology. 2010;75(1):112–6.
7. Kuo YC, Liu SP, Chen JH, Chang HC, Tsai VF, Hsieh JT. Feasibility of a novel audio-video sexual stimulation system: an adjunct to the use of penile duplex Doppler ultrasonography for the investigation of erectile dysfunction. J Sex Med. 2010;7(12):3979–83.
8. Caretta N, Palego P, Roverato A, Selice R, Ferlin A, Foresta C. Age-matched cavernous peak systolic velocity: a highly sensitive parameter in the diagnosis of arteriogenic erectile dysfunction. Int J Impot Res. 2006;18(3):306.
9. Lue TF, Hricak H, Marich K, Tanagho E. Vasculogenic impotence evaluated by high-resolution ultrasonography and pulsed Doppler spectrum analysis. Radiology. 1985;155(3):777–81.
10. Meuleman EJ, Hatzichristou D, Rosen RC, Sadovsky R. Diagnostic tests for male erectile dysfunction revisited. J Sex Med. 2010;7(7):2375–81.
11. Ghafoori M, Hoseini K, Shakiba M. Comparison of one-side and bilateral intracavernosal papaverine injection on a Doppler study of the penis. Int J Impot Res. 2009;21(6):382.
12. Pagano MJ, Stahl PJ. Variation in penile hemodynamics by anatomic location of cavernosal artery imaging in penile duplex Doppler ultrasound. J Sex Med. 2015;12(9):1911–9.
13. Radparvar JR, Lim G, Chiem AT. Effect of insonation angle on peak systolic velocity variation. Am J Emerg Med. 2020;38(2):173–7.
14. Chung E, De Young L, Brock GB. Penile duplex ultrasonography in men with Peyronie's disease: is it veno-occlusive dysfunction or poor cavernosal arterial inflow that contributes to erectile dysfunction? J Sex Med. 2011;8(12):3446–51.
15. Bönhof JA, McLaughlin G. Artifacts in sonography–Part 3. Ultraschall Med. 2018;39(3):260–83.
16. Hügel U, Rosenov A, Baumgartner I, Thalhammer C. Vascular color-coded duplex ultrasound in practice: artifacts. Praxis. 2019;108(10):679–84.

Chapter 14
Limitations of Penile Hemodynamic Studies with Doppler Ultrasound

14.1 Introduction

Penile Doppler ultrasound (PDU) has emerged as a valuable tool for assessing penile vascular health and diagnosing erectile dysfunction (ED) [1]. However, as with any diagnostic technique, PDU is not without limitations. Understanding the limitations of PDU is essential for clinicians, researchers, and healthcare practitioners who utilize this technique for evaluating erectile function. By acknowledging the boundaries of PDU studies, practitioners can make informed decisions, accurately interpret results, and develop comprehensive treatment plans that encompass both the strengths and weaknesses of this diagnostic modality.

14.2 The Paradox of Normal Versus Abnormal in PDU Studies

PDU studies often present a paradoxical challenge when it comes to distinguishing between normal and abnormal hemodynamic findings. While PDU offers valuable insights into penile vascular function, interpreting the significance of the obtained parameters can be intricate and multifaceted [2].

Defining what constitutes a "normal" hemodynamic parameter in PDU studies is not always straightforward. It is a fact that the most common cutoffs (PSV > 30 cm/s and EDV < 5 cm/s) will not yield an accuracy of 100%, meaning that some patients outside this limit may eventually be in the normal spectrum [3]. Perhaps a patient with bilateral PSVs of 31 cm/s will not have a different outcome from another man with PSV of 29 cm/s, though one will be classified as normal and the other not according to the standardization suggested in this book. Therefore, we suggest that

© The Author(s), under exclusive license to Springer Nature
Switzerland AG 2024
E. d. P. Miranda, F. Carneiro, *Penile Color Duplex-Doppler Ultrasound in Erectile Dysfunction Diagnosis and Management*,
https://doi.org/10.1007/978-3-031-55649-4_14

borderline values be carefully interpreted. In case of doubt, normalcy should be favored, as abnormal reports may have a severe and detrimental effect on a patient's perspective of his own condition.

Another relevant issue is the magnitude of blood flow necessary to keep a firm erection may vary significantly according to anatomic patient anatomic characteristics. For example, patients with large penises may require higher inflow to maintain an erection. That is one of the reasons why patients with short penis and borderline low PSVs may have perfectly normal erections. In other words, what may be considered normal in one patient could be indicative of an issue in another, making the determination of normalcy a dynamic and patient-specific process.

14.3 Mixed Vascular Dysfunction of the Penis

PDU often encounter scenarios where the penile vascular dysfunction is not confined to a single etiology. The concept of mixed vascular dysfunction introduces a layer of complexity that challenges the clear distinction between arterial insufficiency and CVOD.

Mixed vascular dysfunction refers to cases where both arterial and venous components contribute to ED. The traditional dichotomy between arterial insufficiency and CVOD becomes blurred as patients may exhibit signs of both issues simultaneously. This overlapping pathophysiology poses challenges in attributing symptoms to a single etiology.

Identifying mixed vascular dysfunction solely through PDU studies can be challenging. Some authors advocate some criteria to define the diagnosis of mixed vascular dysfunction when PSV < 25 cm/s, EDV > 6 cm/s, and RI < 0.6 [3]. The authors acknowledge that in the presence of arterial insufficiency, PDU does not have enough specificity to establish the diagnosis of CVOD. For that purpose, an additional dynamic infusion cavernosometry and cavernosography (DICC) would be required for an accurate diagnosis [4]. In such cases, we recommend labeling the patient as plain arterial insufficiency, which is a simple and sound diagnosis and will have the same therapeutic implications.

14.4 Normal Parameters in a Non-responsive Penis

In rigidity-based approach for PDU, assessment of penile rigidity is performed consistently throughout the examination. In most cases, normal hemodynamic parameters are associated an adequate rigidity, ideally >8/10. On the other hand, patients with inadequate rigidity (<6/10; <EHS grade 3) usually display abnormal velocities and Doppler waveforms. However, there are certain scenarios in which clinical radiological dissociation is found.

If during a standard PDU examination after adequate redosing strategy normal parameters are found in a flaccid penis, several hypotheses are plausible. First the examiners must reassure that all US adjustments were adequately performed. It is also important to make sure that it is not a case of loss of sustaining during PDU. As the erection is a dynamic event, it is possible that patient had a good rigidity during Doppler scanning but has progressively loss the erection to a point that during rigidity assessment it was already less rigid. It is important to highlight that PDU is based on flow and resistance parameters to provide an indirect measure of intracavernosal pressure [5]. Therefore, in chronically hypotensive patients, this difference in intracavernosal pressure vs. mean arterial pressure (MAP) may lead to these findings. For example, it is a known fact that intracavernosal pressure of about 90 mmHg generates considerable penile rigidity in normotensive patients (i.e., with blood pressure 120 × 80 mmHg, MAP would be about 90 mmHg) [6, 7]. So if a patient has a MAP of 60 mmHg, lower penile rigidity would eventually lead equivocally to normal parameters and Doppler waveforms, with an estimate intracavernous pressure of 50–60 mmHg. This phenomenon might be suspected with routine measurement of blood pressure prior to PDU examination. And finally, this finding is also possible in patients with distal microangiopathy of vessel and sinusoids, which is eventually seen in decompensated diabetic patients. In these individuals, there is increased arteriolar resistance from distal microvasculature with normal proximal branches of the cavernous arteries, mimicking a high resistance bed, but in reality the erectile tissue is poorly perfused and erection is usually absent. Note that there are multiple complexities and challenges inherent in interpreting these measurements that require expertise and clinical experience.

14.5 Abnormal Parameters in a Hard Penis

As opposed to what was discussed in the previous section, the identification of abnormal parameters in a hard penis is another a possibility during PDU, which also requires careful consideration, given the complexities involved in interpreting these deviations. It is very important to rule out the presence of artifacts or US machine maladjustments such as signal noise, improper probe placement, or reading in vessels outside the corporal bodies. Discerning between genuine abnormalities and artifacts is essential to prevent misdiagnosis. However, if confirmed these aberrations can indicate a compensated dysfunction, which is most found in cases of arterial insufficiency. In other words, in this situation a patient is found with abnormally low PSV values and a rigid erection. This might be possible as a result of either optimal relaxation of penile arteries together with the erectile tissue or compromised development of collateral blood flow to compensate progressive atherosclerosis.

If a patient achieves good clinical response with ICI despite abnormal PDU parameters, this has many implications in his follow-up as he becomes a good candidate for ICI therapy. However, as he already displays signs or arteriopathy and limited blood flow in the main arterial bed, this means that he will eventually have worse prognosis in comparison to those with good ICI response and normal PDU parameters. These subtle distinctions add sophistication when facing with these patients, as opposed to ICI test alone.

14.6   Severe Atherosclerosis in Cavernosal Arteries

The potential challenges and implications of detecting severe atherosclerosis within the cavernosal arteries are evident, highlighting the intricacies that clinicians must navigate when interpreting PDU findings in such cases. Severe atherosclerosis in cavernosal arteries reflects compromised blood flow due to the buildup of atherosclerotic plaques [8]. This condition can significantly impact erectile function by impeding the arterial inflow essential for achieving and maintaining an erection, which will lead to progressive decrease in blood inflow and consequently decrease PSVs and the diagnosis of arterial insufficiency. The main limitation in this scenario is when in obstruction might generate multiple stenotic points and capturing the real velocities in the cavernosal arteries may become challenging. Also, post-stenotic acceleration in cavernosal arteries may occur, which is a phenomenon that can potentially mimic normal vascular conditions. This acceleration occurs when blood flow encounters a stenotic or narrowed segment in the artery. Beyond the stenosis, the blood flow accelerates as it passes through the narrowed region, resulting in increased velocity readings downstream. This can lead to falsely elevated PSV. Consequently, in cases where post-stenotic acceleration is present, the PDU scanning might indicate apparently normal blood flow parameters. Careful consideration of this phenomenon is crucial during the interpretation of penile Doppler ultrasound studies to avoid misdiagnosis or overlooking potential underlying vascular issues. It is very important that the examiner searches for a clean segment of at least 1 cm without the presence of post-stenotic acceleration in the proximal aspect of the cavernosal bodies, which can be challenging and eventually impossible. In addition, there are some cases with complete occlusion of the cavernosal artery that will not allow the identification of a reliable PSV, in which the distal vascular bed is filled by collateral circulation. When that is the case, the authors recommend that a descriptive analysis be provided instead of trying to find a reliable PSV, as it may not always capture the subtleties of arterial plaques, especially in cases of deep-seated or calcified lesions.

14.7   Geometric Erectile Dysfunction

The concept of geometric ED involves the potential problems to axial rigidity that are not a result of penile hemodynamics. In fact, an adequate blood flow will ensure radial rigidity, but axial rigidity involves other principles such as penile geometry and biomechanical properties of the tunica albuginea [9]. Although PDU studies provide valuable insights into the hemodynamic aspects of ED, when confronted with geometric ED, the limitations of PDU become evident.

Geometric ED refers to alterations in the penile shape or geometry that impede proper erectile function [10]. This condition can encompass penile deformities, fibrotic changes, or structural anomalies that affect the ability to achieve a rigid and functional erection. While PDU excels at assessing blood flow dynamics, it may encounter limitations in characterizing the structural aspects of geometric ED. Moreover, PDU usually evaluates blood inflow through the proximal aspect of the cavernosal bodies, while some patients with Peyronie's disease (PD) have distal distortions of the tunica albuginea that will impact tissue expansion in that area. In such cases, patients might display normal PDU parameters with adequate proximal rigidity, but the distal shaft will not engorge as expected. PDU examiners should be fully aware of this limitation, as PDU primarily focuses on hemodynamics and may not capture the nuances of fibrotic or structural changes responsible for the geometric abnormalities. These situations indicate severe PD with significant negative consequences on erectile function and will require more invasive treatment strategies, similarly to those with primary abnormal PDU parameters [11].

14.8 Using Clinical Parameters to Solve Potential Limitations

Navigating the limitations of PDU studies requires a comprehensive approach that integrates clinical parameters to complement the information obtained from hemodynamic assessments, which emphasizes the importance of context-driven interpretation. An abnormal hemodynamic parameter in isolation may not always signify a pathological condition. Patient-specific factors, such as anxiety, medications, or even recent sexual activity, can transiently influence PDU readings. Contextual interpretation is crucial to avoid overdiagnosis and overtreatment based solely on abnormal PDU findings.

Integrating PDU findings with the patient's medical history, physical examination, and other diagnostic modalities is the key to overcome all PDU limitations. When in doubt, repeating PDU assessment may shed light on the controversial issues. At all times, PDU findings must be in accordance to patient' history and pretest probabilities, so that clinical judgment ensures a balanced approach to diagnosis and treatment decisions.

14.9 Conclusions

The limitations inherent to PDU underscore the need for a nuanced approach to interpreting findings and making clinical decisions. This chapter explored the complexities of navigating these limitations and highlighted the importance of integrating clinical parameters to ensure accurate diagnoses. Embracing nuance and recognizing the limitations of PDU is the first step toward overcoming these limitations. The intricate interplay between hemodynamics, structural aspects, and patient-specific factors demands a thorough understanding that extends beyond the scope of PDU alone. This highlights the importance of incorporating other conceptual and contextual factors to enrich diagnostic accuracy and guide treatment decisions. Ultimately, the insights gained from this chapter emphasize that while PDU has its limitations, it remains an essential tool in diagnosing and managing erectile dysfunction when complemented by a thorough clinical assessment and a multidisciplinary approach.

References

1. Nashed A, Lokeshwar SD, Frech F, Mann U, Patel P. The efficacy of penile duplex ultrasound in erectile dysfunction management decision-making: a systematic review. Sex Med Rev. 2021;9(3):472–7.
2. Carneiro F, Saito OC, Miranda EP. Standardization of penile hemodynamic evaluation through color duplex-doppler ultrasound. Rev Assoc Med Bras (1992). 2020;66(9):1180–6.
3. Sikka SC, Hellstrom WJ, Brock G, Morales AM. Standardization of vascular assessment of erectile dysfunction: standard operating procedures for duplex ultrasound. J Sex Med. 2013;10(1):120–9.
4. Gao QQ, Chen JH, Chen Y, Song T, Dai YT. Dynamic infusion cavernosometry and cavernosography for classifying venous erectile dysfunction and its significance for individual treatment. Chin Med J. 2019;132(4):405–10.
5. Lue TF. Erectile dysfunction. N Engl J Med. 2000;342(24):1802–13.
6. Hsu GL, Hung YP, Tsai MH, Chang HC, Liu SP, Molodysky E, et al. The venous drainage of the corpora cavernosa in the human penis. Arab J Urol. 2013;11(4):384–91.
7. Mulhall JP, Damaser MS. Development of a mathematical model for the prediction of the area of venous leak. Int J Impot Res. 2001;13(4):236–9.
8. Warboys CM, Amini N, de Luca A, Evans PC. The role of blood flow in determining the sites of atherosclerotic plaques. F1000 Med Rep. 2011;3:5.
9. Udelson D. Biomechanics of male erectile function. J R Soc Interface. 2007;4(17):1031–47.
10. Pescatori ES, Drei B, Silingardi V. Advanced diagnostics in erectile dysfunction: beyond the concept of hemodynamics. J Endocrinol Invest. 2003;26(3 Suppl):125–6.
11. Nehra A, Alterowitz R, Culkin DJ, Faraday MM, Hakim LS, Heidelbaugh JJ, et al. Peyronie's disease: AUA guideline. J Urol. 2015;194(3):745–53.

Chapter 15
Applicability of Additional Penile Investigation Modalities Using Ultrasound Devices

15.1 Introduction

Because of its superior image quality, lack of ionizing radiation, relative portability, and low cost, ultrasound (US) is the imaging modality of choice for a wide range of clinical purposes. Over the past few decades, there have been numerous technological advancements in US technology, including color and power Doppler, speckle reduction, compound imaging, harmonic imaging, and 3D imaging, all of which have become the norm of care and added crucial data to US examinations. Elastography, microvascular imaging, and US contrast media have all recently entered clinical usage [1]. This chapter will demonstrate how these new tools can be used to assess the penile in the context of sexual medicine.

15.2 Elastography

Manual palpation has been a cornerstone of physical diagnosis for centuries, ever since the first physicians realized that disease processes undetectable to the human sight could frequently be detected by their firmness. This difference in tissue hardness or rigidity between sick and healthy tissue is the foundation of elasticity imaging. In addition to B-mode imaging and Doppler imaging, elasticity imaging adds stiffness as a third tissue feature to the US arsenal for lesion diagnosis and characterization. Elastography is based on the assumption that palpable abnormalities, such as cancer or other pathologies, are typically "harder" (less elastic) than normal tissue [2]. US can determine the relative stiffness of a lesion using a variety of approaches that exploit tissue features and the interplay between sound and extrinsic compression.

© The Author(s), under exclusive license to Springer Nature Switzerland AG 2024
E. d. P. Miranda, F. Carneiro, *Penile Color Duplex-Doppler Ultrasound in Erectile Dysfunction Diagnosis and Management*,
https://doi.org/10.1007/978-3-031-55649-4_15

Penile ultrasonography is a well-established imaging technique used in sexual medicine. With high-resolution ultrasound probes, the anatomy of the penis may be studied in great detail, and cavernosal hemodynamics can be evaluated using spectral Doppler analysis. In 1981, Gelbard et al. reported using ultrasound to evaluate plaques in Peyronie's disease (PD) for the first time in the medical literature [3]. In 1985, Lue et al. assessed vasculogenic erectile dysfunction (ED) using high-resolution ultrasonography and pulsed Doppler spectrum analysis [4]. Since then, technologic improvements in imaging quality, portability, and new operational modes have emerged in ultrasound imaging, expanding its utility in medicine. Elastography is an example of these improvements and consists of a noninvasive ultrasound imaging modality for evaluating tissue stiffness [5]. Basically, it can be operated according to two different methodologies: strain elastography (SE) and shear wave elastography (SWE). SE is a semiquantitative method in which repetitive compressions are applied with the transducer. Tissue mobility in the scanned area after mechanical compression generates different signals according to tissue elasticity and is translated in a color box [5]. Because it relies on manual skill to produce consistent results, SE produces more variable results. SWE, on the other hand, is a quantitative technique that uses acoustic impulses to cause molecular vibrations within the tissue. Because elasticity is related to the speed of the waves, the vibrations that induce them produce shear waves, which may then be used to compute elasticity. Kilopascals or centimeters per second are two ways to express these measurements [6]. Kilopascal is a unit for measuring pressure that is used to determine internal stress, elastic modulus, and eventually tensile strength. Although this diagnostic method is still very new, it has been advocated for application in a variety of clinical situations. Based on data from meta-analyses, the European Federation of Societies for Ultrasound in Medicine and Biology published guidelines for indications and interpretation patterns of ultrasound elastography [7]. However, most of this evidence is based on experience acquired from liver pathologies, followed by breast, thyroid, gastrointestinal tract, prostate, and musculoskeletal pathologies, in which SE and SWE have proved useful. Interestingly, there are enough data to recommend endoscopic elastography with promising results. Other evaluations such as superficial lymph node assessment, intraoperative brain elastography, uterine cervix evaluation before delivery, testicular tumors, anal incontinence, arterial plaque stiffness, and others were not included because of insufficient data at the time of publication [8].

In sexual medicine, quantifying changes in erectile tissue stiffness might be useful, particularly in circumstances where the onset of cavernous fibrosis is a frequent indicator of disease progression [8]. Fewer smooth muscle cells and alterations in collagen structure in the cavernous bodies have been described in ED, PD, aging, testosterone deficiency, and priapism. Moreover, identification of diffuse areas of abnormal erectile tissue elasticity could predict higher doses of intracavernosal agents to achieve an erection or even be a target for antifibrotic therapy. Rigidity assessment is another application for elastography, because increments in intracavernosal pressure after a rigid erection create progressive changes in the elastic properties of the cavernous bodies and tunica albuginea.

Some preliminary studies have investigated the role of elastography in sexual medicine. Experimental studies were performed in rats comparing SWE values with immunohistochemistry as predictors of penile structural changes [9, 10]. These investigators had similar findings and concluded that SWE can quantitatively and accurately indicate significant changes in the content of collagen fibers and smooth muscle cells within the penis. The feasibility of SWE as a tool for measurement of human cavernous body stiffness was initially investigated in two pilot observational studies [11, 12]. The investigators found SWE to be a reliable tool and found a significant correlation between SWE figures and age [11, 12], or sex hormone levels [12]. A controlled study suggested that SWE might aid in the diagnosis of ED, regardless of etiology [13]. The investigators analyzed 70 patients and found that, compared with control subjects, patients with ED had lower SWE values. The cutoff value of 17.1 kPa yielded a specificity of 95% and a positive predictive value of 85% for the diagnosis of moderate to severe ED [13].

In the radical prostatectomy population, elastography could be particularly helpful because it is believed that cavernous nerve injury during surgery might lead to penile collagenation. In theory, it would be useful in the diagnosis and follow-up of initial fibrotic tissue change in the cavernous bodies. A recent prospective study investigated 65 patients who underwent open radical prostatectomy with different nerve-sparing techniques [14]. The investigators found that elasticity figures had a strong correlation with International Index of Erectile Function scores.

Elastography also has been used in the evaluation of patients with structural changes in the tunica albuginea such as those found in patients with PD. Riversi et al. [15] found that SE improved the accuracy of B-mode ultrasound in detecting plaques in the tunica albuginea. Richards et al. [16] reported on a case of PD with non-palpable plaque and severe curvature. This plaque could not be identified on B-mode ultrasonography, and SWE identified an area close to the point of maximum curvature where injection therapy could be performed.

In addition, it has been suggested that SWE also might be useful as a surrogate for Erection Hardness Scale (EHS) scores during Doppler ultrasound studies in patients with ED and curvature assessments for PD. Yang et al. [17] showed that tunica albuginea elasticity measured by SWE during induced erection correlates with EHS scores. This finding is relevant and could be of clinical utility, because assessing rigidity and measuring Doppler velocities of the cavernous arteries simultaneously can be very challenging. A more recent study by Zhang et al. (10) showed a significant association between elastography values and responsiveness to erectogenic medication in patients with ED.

Virtual touch tissue quantification (VTTQ) is an elastography protocol that measures the mean shear wave velocities (SWV) of cavernous bodies and glans in the transverse and longitudinal planes. It has been described as a method that can evaluate penile rigidity and can effectively and sensitively indicate the axial and radial rigidity changes in penile erection [18, 19]. It is possible to assume that SWV is proportional to tissue rigidity. SWV is fundamentally correlated with the main mechanical properties indicating material rigidity, assuming the material is linear, isotropic, and elastic. The more rigid the tissue, the more rapidly the shear wave will propagate. However, those studies showed that as erection grades increased, SWV values decreased; that is, the firmer the penis, the slower the shear wave propagated. There were a negative correlation between SWV and penile rigidity [19]. This observation can be explained by the fact that the cavernous body of the penis is not a linear, isotropic, elastic body and that the penile erection is a result of multiple neurovascular events. Therefore, we believe that tunica albuginea stiffness evaluation is more reliable than the cavernous bodies stiffness evaluation since it is more isotropic, linear, and elastic [17]. Another important issue is that longitudinal and transverse ultrasound cavernous body images and their measurements of stiffness probably do not correlate directly to axial and radial rigidities. This assumption derives from the complexity of the concepts involved in penile rigidity and the fact that the tunica albuginea, which is an integral responsible for the rigidity phenomenon, was not routinely included in the measurements of the studies that proposed this methodology.

There is no described contraindication for performing elastography. It does not apply ionizing radiation, and safety recommendations are the same as those of conventional ultrasound imaging modes. In addition, it is acceptable to patients because it is noninvasive and can be easily performed in a regular ultrasound examination room [8]. The learning curve for experts in penile ultrasonography is expected to be very low because the technique is virtually identical to conventional ultrasound. SWE is not affected by section selection, which makes it even more convenient to examiners.

However, this method has some limitations. SWE signals require a minimum distance between the targeted area and the probe, which might be difficult because penile internal structures do not have large dimensions. Also, a limited number of areas of interest are captured per study and more inelastic are as might not be captured in cases with heterogeneous fibrotic changes. Moreover, it is more time consuming than plain ultrasonography and requires specific training. To our knowledge, there are no publications that assess the intra- and interobserver variabilities for these two methods of penile elastography. In addition, fibrosis is a spectrum rather than a categorical entity, and the minimum requirements of tissue elasticity for proper penile function remain unknown. Therefore, to optimize outcomes in clinical practice by decreasing variability and cofounding factors, this diagnostic procedure should be performed in a standardized fashion. SWE should be preferably used over SE because the latter depends on the ability of the performer to routinely maintain the same compression magnitude. In other words, SWE is easier to perform and provides less artifactual images. Transducers must be ideally applied as close as possible to the area of interest, with a distance of no more than 3–4 cm. Because the penis is a mobile anatomic structure, steady fixation is strongly recommended to decrease slippery movements that might generate inaccurate numbers. Readings in areas of calcification should be avoided in the tunica albuginea and cavernosal bodies. Calcium deposits are prevalent in penile ultrasonography and might overestimate tissue stiffness. Inflammatory skin alterations also can change the elastographic pattern, and such areas should not be chosen whenever possible [8].

The fact is there has been no accurate and noninvasive way to measure structural cavernous body changes in clinical practice, and elastography has the potential to fill this gap in the future. This assessment is relevant and might aid clinicians in predicting treatment outcomes and in preparing for surgery, particularly in the aforementioned conditions with high risk for penile fibrosis. Despite the known limitations and the sparse literature available, we believe elastography, especially SWE, is a very promising diagnostic tool in sexual medicine and should be further evaluated. Significant developments in ultrasound technology are expected and will improve imaging quality, ease of use, quantification, and range of tissue characteristics that are measurable using SWE. Development of a standard of practice and accurate cutoff levels that are clinically meaningful are warranted before it can become a universally accepted tool for the assessment of erectile tissue elasticity.

15.3 Contrast-Enhanced Ultrasound Imaging (CEUS)

Due to the inherent contrast disparities between solid tissues and blood, US imaging uses the echoes produced by sound waves interacting with tissues to create 2- or 3D anatomical pictures that enable the differentiation of macrovasculature from organs without the need of contrast agents. Doppler imaging is highly accurate at detecting and quantifying blood flow in large vessels with high-velocity blood flow, but it is not able to detect flow in capillaries or smaller veins. Due to the introduction of microbubbles (MBs) as contrast agents for US, it is now possible to identify images of microscopic vessels with low-velocity flows [20]. This is made possible by MBs' capacity to scatter acoustic waves and the distinctive harmonics that they produce when subjected to ultrasound. This makes it possible to visualize the vasculature in real time with excellent spatial resolution and safety without using ionizing radiation.

MBs are tiny (1–4 mm) gas-liquid emulsions formed of a stabilizer shell made of biocompatible materials enclosing a gas core. Due to their small size, MBs remain contained to the vasculature after injection into a peripheral vein, including microcapillaries, and can be detected in circulation for a period of time ranging from a few minutes to 60 min. This duration usually depends on their composition, method of injection, and dose, before their gas core diffuses out of the shell and the components are eliminated by the reticuloendothelial system [21]. In many different tissues, such as the heart, liver, spleen, bowel, pancreas, kidneys, breast, ovaries, and prostate, this time frame is sufficient to gather meaningful information on vascularity, perfusion rates, and potential tumor detection. In the heart, contrast-enhanced ultrasound (CEUS) has been utilized to locate atherosclerotic carotid plaques that are at risk for rupture and to enhance imaging of artery wall abnormalities [22]. Although MB has been widely used in the liver for clinical lesion detection, it has also proved successful at detecting masses in other organs such as the kidney, pancreas, ovaries, and prostate [20]. Due to the vascular makeup of localized liver lesions, variations in the filling time and washout of the MB contrast agent can make it easier to characterize focal lesions in addition to identifying them from the surrounding tissue [23].

The molecular targeting of the MB contrast agents, which enables not only the detection of anatomical and circulatory structures but also the imaging of biological processes like angiogenesis and inflammation, is another interesting area for CEUS applications. The protective shell of MBs can be combined with a targeting peptide, receptor ligand, or antibody to enable them to bind and accumulate in regions expressing the complementary protein. This is known as molecular targeting of MBs. Proangiogenic factors, such as VEGFR2, endoglin, and integrin v3, have been used to target, visualize, and monitor angiogenesis. P-selectin or mucosal address in cellular adhesion molecule (MadCAM), which are used to target and monitor inflammation, are some of the targets being investigated [20].

There is only one known study pertaining to the use of CEUS in diagnosing venous erectile dysfunction [24]. Forty-six individuals underwent cavernosography, and 23 of them were diagnosed with venous leakage. These patients then received cavernous injection and CEUS injection, and CEUS validated the diagnosis of venous leakage in 21 patients. In addition, CEUS was able to identify possible locations of more intense leak and distinguished between patients with double venous leak, single venous leak, crural venous leak, and mixed venous leak. The authors advocated that CEUS could be considered accurate, safe, and less invasive in diagnosing venous leak in the penis [24].

In conclusion, CEUS is a low-cost, safe clinical imaging technique that has the potential to identify and characterize pathologies by allowing patients to see how their tissue is perfused and vascularized. Improvements in 3D US will likely increase its dependability while also making it more practical for use in clinics. With the most recent preclinical advancements in the molecular targeting of MBs, CEUS could be combined with other imaging modalities for the most accurate illness detection and tracking. Regarding CEUS usage in sexual medicine, the literature on this topic is very limited, but the potential future use of CEUS to investigate ED seems promising.

15.4   Microvascular Imaging

As mentioned earlier in this chapter, the main imaging technique used in clinical practice to evaluate morphological changes in human tissues and organs, particularly superficial lesions, is US imaging. However, it might still be challenging to identify severe illnesses in some cases and to monitor small changes in lesions using standard US [25]. Blood flow is a crucial evaluation criterion for lesions among other features, since angiogenesis is an essential aspect in the development and progression of malignancies, and the growth of tumors depends on the production and expansion of aberrant blood vessels. A common indicator of neovascularity in tumors on sonography, which is frequently used to diagnose a variety of malignancies, is the distribution of vessels. Power Doppler flow imaging (PD) and color

Doppler flow imaging (CD) are two popular techniques for illustrating blood flow in lesions; however, it might be challenging to fully understand low velocity blood flow. Contrast-enhanced ultrasonography (CEUS) can make it easier to assess the tumor's blood supply and provide perfusion data, which may enhance diagnostic performance (as seen in CEUS section). However, the application may be constrained by the invasive fashion of MB contrasts and the associated high costs. Microvascular flow imaging (MFI) shows blood flow on the B-scan picture in real time [26]. The considerably weaker echoes of blood cells may be seen as a result of the methodology which echoes are recorded, processed, and filtered. These weaker echoes are shown as a flow by comparing succeeding frames. To varied degrees, manufacturers have currently implemented this technology. The benefits include a noticeably higher spatial resolution that is comparable to that of B-scan sonography and a better representation of slow flow with fewer artifacts than CD. Microflow imaging is anticipated to increasingly supplement CD without replacing it in the future due to constraints including the absence of velocity measurement and penetration depth [27]. Other possibilities for MFI use are to enhance conventional Doppler ultrasound methods with improved filters and faster frame rates to improve the separation of background noise from slow-moving signals. These cutting-edge Doppler methods go by names like microvascular imaging (MVI) (Philips Medical Systems) or superb microvascular imaging (SMI) (Canon Medical Systems). The developing Doppler ultrasound technology superb microvascular imaging (SMI) improves the diagnostic effectiveness of traditional grayscale US by delineating a wider spectrum of blood flow patterns with higher resolution. In the last several years, there has been a tremendous advancement in the use of SMI in other organs such as thyroid, breast, lymph nodes, and testis. SMI can be used to show the distribution of blood flow as well as the number of microvessels, which can give clinicians more specific information regarding lesions. In rare circumstances, SMI may even be used in place of CEUS to diagnose a great number of different illnesses and assess the effectiveness of their treatment.

At the time of publishing this book, only one study has investigated the utility of SMI in the diagnosis of penile vascular erectile dysfunction [28]. Seventy-two individuals with previously identified vascular ED were assessed using CD and SMI. SMI was able to demonstrate blood flow grades in patients with vascular ED faster and more accurately than conventional CD. They found that SMI is superior to CD because it better depicts the blood flow of the penile cavernous artery and shortens the duration of the test; therefore, it justifies broad usage in the diagnosis of vascular ED.

MFI has also been considered superior to other noninvasive microvessel examination techniques. Patients can benefit from this efficient and cost-effective solution. Moreover, it is important to mention that pathological analysis using histologic microvessel density is another possibility to evaluate actual blood perfusion of tissues and organs. However, even such invasive evaluation has not been considered more effective than MFI in detecting the number and location of blood vessels. The most relevant disadvantages of MFI approaches are their lack of directionality and the fact that MFI may also have a diminished effect on deeper organs.

15.5   Conclusion

Numerous new ultrasound technologies are currently being developed and launched to the market, with the potential to significantly expand sonography's capabilities. Elastrography, CEUS, and microvascular flow imaging are some of the new features with potential increasing use in sexual medicine that might be used to evaluate hemodynamics and mechanical properties of the penile shaft.

References

1. Abdo CHN, Oliveira WM Jr, Moreira Junior ED, Fittipaldi JAS. Perfil sexual da população brasileira: resultados do Estudo do Comportamento Sexual (ECOS) do Brasileiro. Rev Bras Med. 2002;59:250–7.
2. Ophir J, Cespedes I, Ponnekanti H, Yazdi Y, Li X. Elastography: a quantitative method for imaging the elasticity of biological tissues. Ultrason Imaging. 1991;13(2):111–34.
3. Gelbard M, Sarti D, Kaufman J. Ultrasound imaging of Peyronie's plaques. J Urol. 1981;125(1):44–6.
4. Lue TF, Hricak H, Marich K, Tanagho E. Vasculogenic impotence evaluated by high-resolution ultrasonography and pulsed Doppler spectrum analysis. Radiology. 1985;155(3):777–81.
5. Arda K, Ciledag N, Aktas E, Arıbas BK, Köse K. Quantitative assessment of normal soft-tissue elasticity using shear-wave ultrasound elastography. Am J Roentgenol. 2011;197(3):532–6.
6. DeWall RJ. Ultrasound elastography: principles, techniques, and clinical applications. Crit Rev Biomed Eng. 2013;41(1):1–19.
7. Cosgrove D, Piscaglia F, Bamber J, Bojunga J, Correas J-M, Gilja O, et al. EFSUMB guidelines and recommendations on the clinical use of ultrasound elastography. Part 2: clinical applications. Ultraschall Med. 2013;34(03):238–53.
8. Carneiro F, Miranda EP. Penile elastography: current and future applications in sexual medicine. J Sex Med. 2018;15(6):816–9.
9. Qiao X, Zhang J, Gao F, Li F, Liu Y, Xing L, et al. An experimental study: evaluating the tissue structure of penis with 2D-ShearWave™ Elastography. Int J Impot Res. 2017;29(1):12.
10. Zhang J, Qiao X, Gao F, Li F, Bai M, Zhang H, et al. A new method of measuring the stiffness of corpus cavernosum penis with ShearWave™ Elastography. Br J Radiol. 2015;88(1048):20140671.
11. Inci E, Turkay R, Nalbant MO, Yenice MG, Tugcu V. The value of shear wave elastography in the quantification of corpus cavernosum penis rigidity and its alteration with age. Eur J Radiol. 2017;89:106–10.
12. Zhang J-J, Qiao X-H, Gao F, Bai M, Li F, Du L-F, et al. Smooth muscle cells of penis in the rat: noninvasive quantification with shear wave elastography. Biomed Res Int. 2015;2015:595742.
13. Turkay R, Inci E, Yenice MG, Tugcu V. Shear wave elastography: can it be a new radiologic approach for the diagnosis of erectile dysfunction? Ultrasound. 2017;25(3):150–5.
14. Hamidi N, Altinbas N, Gokce M, Suer E, Yagci C, Baltaci S, et al. Preliminary results of a new tool to evaluate cavernous body fibrosis following radical prostatectomy: penile elastography. Andrology. 2017;5(5):999–1006.
15. Riversi V, Tallis V, Trovatelli S, Belba A, Volterrani L, Iacoponi F, et al. Realtime-elastosonography of the penis in patients with Peyronie's disease. Arch Ital Urol Androl. 2012;84:174–7.
16. Richards G, Goldenberg E, Pek H, Gilbert BR. Penile sonoelastography for the localization of a non-palpable, non-sonographically visualized lesion in a patient with penile curvature from Peyronie's disease. J Sex Med. 2014;11(2):516–20.

17. Yang L, Cheng H, Ruan L. MP84-15 a new method of quantitatively measuring penile erection hardness in erectile dysfunction patients: real-time ultrasonic shear wave elastography. J Urol. 2017;197(4):e1145.
18. Rohrer GE, Premo H, Lentz AC. Current techniques for the objective measures of erectile hardness. Sex Med Rev. 2022;10:648.
19. Zheng X, Ji P, Mao H, Wu J. Evaluation of penile erection rigidity in healthy men using virtual touch tissue quantification. Radiol Oncol. 2012;46(2):114–8.
20. Claudon M, Cosgrove D, Albrecht T, Bolondi L, Bosio M, Calliada F, et al. Guidelines and good clinical practice recommendations for contrast enhanced ultrasound (CEUS)-update 2008. Ultraschall Med. 2008;29(1):28–44.
21. Correas J-M, Bridal L, Lesavre A, Méjean A, Claudon M, Hélénon O. Ultrasound contrast agents: properties, principles of action, tolerance, and artifacts. Eur Radiol. 2001;11(8):1316–28.
22. Solbiati L, Martegani A, Leen E. Contrast-enhanced ultrasound of liver diseases. Springer Science & Business Media; 2003.
23. Solbiati L, Martegani A, Leen E, Correas JM, Burns PN, Becker D, et al. Contrast ultrasound technology. In: Contrast-enhanced ultrasound of liver diseases; 2003. p. 1–19.
24. Gao Q-Q, Jin Z-B, Shi L, Chen Y, Chen H, Yu W, et al. Contrast-enhanced ultrasonography in the diagnosis of venous erectile dysfunction. Zhonghua Nan Ke Xue. 2017;23(7):626–9.
25. Li Q, Hu M, Chen Z, Li C, Zhang X, Song Y, et al. Meta-analysis: contrast-enhanced ultrasound versus conventional ultrasound for differentiation of benign and malignant breast lesions. Ultrasound Med Biol. 2018;44(5):919–29.
26. Bonacchi G, Becciolini M, Seghieri M. Superb microvascular imaging: a potential tool in the detection of FNH. J Ultrasound. 2017;20(2):179–80.
27. Fu Z, Zhang J, Lu Y, Wang S, Mo X, He Y, et al. Clinical applications of superb microvascular imaging in the superficial tissues and organs: a systematic review. Acad Radiol. 2021;28(5):694–703.
28. Lan X-F, Jiang F, Peng M, Wu T-T, Xie X, Wu J, et al. Application of superb microvascular imaging in manifesting the blood flow of the penile cavernous artery in vascular ED patients. Zhonghua Nan Ke Xue. 2019;25(3):238–42.

Chapter 16
Optimizing Written Medical Reports

16.1   Introduction

Structured reporting (SR) of ultrasound examinations can be very beneficial for examiners, patient, and the medical team responsible for patient care and is considered a very helpful tool in the field of radiology. Reports could be produced more quickly, more accurately, and more clearly. It aids in the process of communicating with patients and referring to colleagues. Consistent descriptive data can also facilitate institution-based cooperation and research [1].

Generally, SR can be divided into three stages of increasing standardization, in which the highest stage includes the extensive use of structured language [2, 3]. Generally, the report is divided into sections pertaining to methodology, clinical history, findings, and the radiologist's impression or conclusion using headings in the simplest form. In ultrasound examinations, all of these details may be useful. SR can improve the efficiency with which an ultrasound report is generated. In other words, using SR will facilitate the process of writing reports, in which the examiner will just need to revise the anatomical abnormality descriptors, complete the measurements, and provide an impression. Overall, it is the authors understanding that a good report has a clear standard language and uniform presentation of essential, necessary data. Contrary to unclear and verbose reports, structured reports might emphasize simple style and terminology to promote understanding and use of specialized terms to increase clarity [4, 5]. Referring providers do in fact believe SR to be clearer than freestyle ones [6]. When it comes to penile Doppler ultrasound (PDU), we believe that choosing the right amount of information is essential.

SR can also help with research and collaboration among different institutions by using structured components, such as shared common data elements or standard language [4, 7]. Since they have been advocated for more than 10 years, structured reports have grown in popularity and acceptability throughout radiology [8].

© The Author(s), under exclusive license to Springer Nature Switzerland AG 2024

E. d. P. Miranda, F. Carneiro, *Penile Color Duplex-Doppler Ultrasound in Erectile Dysfunction Diagnosis and Management*, https://doi.org/10.1007/978-3-031-55649-4_16

16.2 Structured Report Template for Penile Hemodynamic Evaluation

16.2.1 Methodology

It is critical to explain the study's approach. For instance, a high-frequency linear probe is generally used to perform penile scanning both in the flaccid state and during an erection. We recommend that a brief description of probe in terms of brand and frequency provided by the manufacturer be included in the report.

16.2.2 Clinical Findings

The report should ideally begin with brief clinical information regarding the patient's history and physical exam. Diseases, prescriptions, prior erectile dysfunction drug use, and best quality erection (BQE) at home are important piece of information and could be included in initial statement of the report.

16.2.3 B-Mode Sonographic Findings

The epidermis and subcutaneous tissue should be described first, followed by the spongiosal body, tunica albuginea, and cavernous bodies. Any abnormal or unusual findings of these structures must be reported, which include but are not limited to heterogeneity, hyperechoic regions, and plaques both calcified or non-calcified.

Cavernous arteries could be described in detail. Tortuosity, calcifications, medio-intimal complex thickening, stenotic spots, and obstructions must all be cited. Anatomical variations, the presence of early bifurcations, or multiple cavernosal arteries should also be mentioned [9].

16.2.4 Pharmacological Induction and Reversion Schedule

After pertinent patient history and anatomical description, the erection induction protocol using vasoactive drugs should be specified. A description of the vasoactive agent with the exact substance concentrations and dosage must be recorded. If redosing strategy is necessary, a description of the number of injections and the volume of each injection should be ideally provided. The same concept applies for the need of erection reversal: the description of the sympathomimetic agent, dilution, and number of doses is also a valuable piece of information and should be included in the report.

16.2.5 *Audiovisual Sexual Stimulation*

Since it has been reported that the utilization audiovisual sexual stimulation (AVSS) may reduce patient anxiety and the need of redosing of erectogenic medication, it has become an important step of standardized PDU examinations. The bedroom setting created by this may result in more accurate hemodynamic results as it facilitates total relaxation of the smooth muscles of the cavernous body [10]. Failure to provide AVSS because of patient refusal might eventually have clinical implications. Therefore, we suggest that the utilization of AVSS should also be routinely included in the report.

16.2.6 *Hemodynamic Parameters*

Traditional PDU reports usually include multiple measures of hemodynamic parameters that are eventually measured in time-based protocol in 5, 10, 15, and eventually 20 min. Our understanding is that the most relevant measure is the one obtained during the peak of penile rigidity. Although multiple time points may eventually be informed in the report with the intent of providing a more detailed description, we advocate that it might become confusing. Therefore, we suggest that only the best parameters obtained at peak rigidity be provided.

The most common parameters are peak systolic velocity (PSV), ending diastolic velocity (EDV), resistant index (RI), pulsatility index, acceleration, and peak velocity in the dorsal vein, and a few other parameters have been described in the literature. However, they are less important for the final diagnosis and may become a confounding variable as opposed to aiding in the conclusion-drawing process. As our ultimate intent is to simplify and standardize PDU examinations and reports, the author's preference is to inform only the most relevant parameters required for an accurate hemodynamic diagnosis, which are PSVs and EDVs [11]. Though RI values have been classically used for the diagnosis of veno-occlusive dysfunction, they become inaccurate in patients with high PSVs. Therefore, the authors advocate that the reported data should be minimalist, but accurate.

16.2.7 *Rigidity Assessment*

It is mandatory to record the erectile hardness at least at the peak of the erection. This is the most important and challenging observation that should be made during penile hemodynamic examination [11, 12]. The patient's ability to achieve a rigid erection throughout PDU is an important predictive factor for normal penile hemodynamics. Throughout the entire procedure, rigidity must be continuously evaluated, and it is crucial to establish a correlation between rigidity and hemodynamic parameters. In addition, the examiner should evaluate penile axial rigidity manually. We do not recommend patient's self-assessment because it can vary widely based on their psychological state and underestimation of their own hardness. The validated erection hardness score (EHS) and the decimal scale are the recommend ones to assess erection rigidity during PDU [13]. Since the EHS could be easily converted to a decimal scale, with 6/10 (EHS 3) representing the penetration threshold, it is the author's understanding that the decimal scale provides more comprehensible information to patients and providers.

16.2.8 Diagnostic Conclusions and Examiners' Impression

The final diagnosis for hemodynamic parameters should ideally be straightforward. Possible diagnoses include normal penile hemodynamics, unilateral or bilateral arterial insufficiency, or cavernous veno-occlusive dysfunction. Although mixed dysfunction has been described and is defended by renowned authors, it is the authors belief that PDU is not adequately powered for such diagnosis. Moreover, failure to indicate the diagnosis of penile hemodynamic mixed dysfunction as apposed to other abnormal diagnosis will not change patient's treatment or outcome. Additional and significant discoveries may eventually be mentioned briefly as free text in the conclusion. If applicable, a clinical impression may be added as an observation. The authors suggest that these impressions and descriptive comments in the conclusion be limited to a minimum and should be reserved for borderline or inconclusive cases.

16.3 Structured Report Template for Penile Deformity Assessment

Everything described above is also an important aspect in the examination of penile deformities, as hemodynamic assessment of these individuals is fundamental. Therefore, this section will simply provide the additional information to be reported after penile deformity assessments. B-mode sonographic findings and clinical presentation of penile deformities are the most relevant aspects that should be included in PDU reports.

16.3.1 B-Mode Sonographic Findings

Albuginea thickness and calcified plaques in Peyronie's disease must be described as specific B-mode sonographic alterations. Cavernous body ecotexture abnormalities, such as intracavernous microcalcifications, must be documented since they imply more diffuse fibrotic changes. It is important to provide a descriptive comment of the sonographic finding along with location of each alteration such as subcoronal, distal, mid, or proximal in the penile shaft. Delimitation and exact measurement of plaques of extension and depth are possible for more experienced examiners in more sophisticated ultrasound machines. However, the authors recognize that this task might be time-consuming, since Peyronie's disease has been increasingly recognized as a diffuse and heterogeneous condition. It is also a fact that extensive plaque does not necessarily translate into deformity severity or disease stability. Therefore, more general or superficial descriptions for simply indicating the presence and echogenic characteristic of plaque in the tunica albuginea or within the corpora are usually enough for establishing the diagnosis of Peyronie's disease.

16.3.2 Clinical Findings

Clinical examination of penile deformities should be performed both in the flaccid state and during an erection and should be included in the SR of PDU.

Evaluation in the flaccid state should start with clinical history taking, which includes onset of symptoms, pain, palpable abnormalities, and history of penile injuries. Although this initial part is usually not included in the report itself, it is helpful in the conduction of PDU. Palpation of the penile shaft under stretch is essential to allow for the localization of possible plaques. Measurement of stretch flaccid penile length from the pubis to the urethral meatus in centimeters using a firm ruler is recommended and is also a relevant piece of information that should be included in the report.

After inducing and erection with vasoactive agents, it is vital to quantify and classify the deformity. Measures of the angles of curvature, the existence of indentation, penile volume loss with their respective measures, and exact location in the penile shaft must also be reported. Adequate material is required, which usually includes a goniometer, a firm, and a malleable ruler. The examiner must pay full attention to include all the specific details in the report and should not forget to report the deformity nature, magnitude, and location. Each measure should be associated with an indication penile hardness, as rigidity may influence in deformity severity and loss of erection during the exam, which is common, may underestimate disease severity. The distance between the point of maximum curvature and the urethral meatus should also be in the report because it may be helpful in the treatment plan for both surgical cases and those candidates for intralesional therapy. Repeat measures of the penile erect length may be performed if applicable. The evaluation of axial stability defining the presence and the characteristic of instability must be documented and qualified. Photo documentation is worth to be annexed to the report if available and allowed as per institutional policy.

16.3.3   Diagnostic Conclusions and Examiners' Impression

The most important differential diagnoses in the assessment of penile deformities are Peyronie's disease and congenital penile curvature. Therefore, in the conclusion, the examiner must indicate which medical condition was found and also include the diagnosis of penile hemodynamics. As the description in the body of the report usually contains a full description of the deformity, there is no need to repeat everything in the conclusion. If applicable, a clinical impression may be added as an observation.

16.4   Conclusions

Structured reports have many advantages for the ultrasound examiner, the patient, and the referring physician, including faster and more accurate findings, improved communication, better patient care, and easier access to research and standards development. This method of reporting has been adopted and used by radiologists across many institutions, and it is likely to spread throughout other medical specialties who are willing to perform focused ultrasound studies. Therefore, it is very important that PDU examiners are able to provide a structured yet robust description of the most relevant clinical and ultrasonographic findings of penile anatomy and hemodynamics.

References

1. O'Connor SD, Kulkarni NM, Griffin MO Jr, Baruah D, Sudakoff GS, Tolat PP. Structured reporting in ultrasound. Ultrasound Q. 2020;36(1):1–5.
2. Sistrom CL, Langlotz CP. A framework for improving radiology reporting. J Am Coll Radiol. 2005;2(2):159–67.
3. Weiss DL, Langlotz CP. Structured reporting: patient care enhancement or productivity nightmare? Radiology. 2008;249(3):739–47.
4. Bosmans J, Peremans L, Menni M, De Schepper A, Duyck P, Parizel P. Structured reporting: if, why, when, how—and at what expense? Results of a focus group meeting of radiology professionals from eight countries. Insights Imaging. 2012;3(3):295–302.
5. Bosmans JM, Weyler JJ, De Schepper AM, Parizel PM. The radiology report as seen by radiologists and referring clinicians: results of the COVER and ROVER surveys. Radiology. 2011;259(1):184–95.
6. Schwartz LH, Panicek DM, Berk AR, Li Y, Hricak H. Improving communication of diagnostic radiology findings through structured reporting. Radiology. 2011;260(1):174.
7. Rubin DL, Kahn CE Jr. Common data elements in radiology. Radiology. 2017;283(3):837–44.
8. Dunnick NR, Langlotz CP. The radiology report of the future: a summary of the 2007 intersociety conference. J Am Coll Radiol. 2008;5(5):626–9.
9. Tansatit T, Jindarak S, Sampatanukul P, Wannaprasert T. Neurovascular anatomy of the penis and pelvis in Thai males: applications to male-to-female and pelvic surgeries. J Med Assoc Thai. 2007;90(1):121.

10. Carneiro F, Nascimento B, Miranda EP, Cury J, Cerri GG, Chammas MC. Audiovisual sexual stimulation improves diagnostic accuracy of penile doppler ultrasound in patients with erectile dysfunction. J Sex Med. 2020;17(2):249–56.
11. Carneiro F, Saito OC, Miranda EP. Standardization of penile hemodynamic evaluation through color duplex-doppler ultrasound. Rev Assoc Med Bras. 2020;66:1180–6.
12. Nascimento B, Miranda EP, Terrier J-E, Carneiro F, Mulhall JP. A critical analysis of methodology pitfalls in duplex Doppler ultrasound in the evaluation of patients with erectile dysfunction: technical and interpretation deficiencies. J Sex Med. 2020;17(8):1416–22.
13. Mulhall JP, Goldstein I, Bushmakin AG, Cappelleri JC, Hvidsten K. Outcomes assessment: validation of the erection hardness score. J Sex Med. 2007;4(6):1626–34.

Chapter 17
Sample of Case Studies

17.1 Introduction

A series of carefully selected case studies are presented in this chapter, each high-lighting a specific clinical scenario and the role of penile Doppler ultrasound in the diagnostic process. These case studies cover a range of conditions, including arterial insufficiency, venous leakage, Peyronie's disease, and normal hemodynamic studies. Each case study provides a comprehensive description of the patient's history, clinical presentation, imaging findings, and subsequent management decisions.

17.2 Case 1

A 31-year-old patient complained of progressive inability to obtain and maintain erection for sexual intercourse for the past 6 months. Two months after the initial presentation, he was started on daily tadalafil 5 mg with a partial and unsatisfactory clinical response. The patient reported that his ED problem began suddenly after a traumatic end of a 2-year relationship. The patient had no significant past medical history and denied concomitant medication use. There was evidence of performance anxiety and low self-esteem. He had no changes in his sexual desire and had preserved morning erections.

Commentary: This is a typical case of a patient with consistent risk factors for psychogenic ED and that may somehow assume that an organic component is also present [1, 2]. PDU studies play an important role in this scenario not only because it aids in ruling out possible organic factors but also has positive therapeutic effects as it demonstrates to the patient that he has anatomical integrity and the ability to have a firm erection. As a result of previous poor sexual experiences, every new

E. d. P. Miranda, F. Carneiro, *Penile Color Duplex-Doppler Ultrasound in
Erectile Dysfunction Diagnosis and Management*,
https://doi.org/10.1007/978-3-031-55649-4_17

sexual encounter is interpreted as stressful, leading to an overactivation of adrenergic pathways that tend to block a rigid erection.

Since this patient had a poor response to PDE5 inhibitors and was interested in a more profound evaluation of his erectile function, a PDU evaluation was scheduled [3]. During the induction protocol, the patients were started with 0.1 mL of standard trimix. After 10 min in his first evaluation, the patient obtained a rigid erection (EHS 4 or 9/10) and scanning was performed. Figures 17.1, 17.2, and 17.3 represent B-mode, color Doppler (CD), and spectral Doppler (PW) evaluations, respectively. The patient was reassessed 1 h after trimix injection and still had a rigid erection (8/10) and received intracavernous etilefrine 10 mg. After 10 min, detumescence was achieved and patient was safely discharged [4–6].

Commentary: During PDU examination, the patient presented normal hemodynamic parameters. These findings are relevant and helpful for the patient to understand and accept his diagnosis of psychogenic ED. The patient was instructed to continue his ED treatment and follow-up with PDE5i and psychotherapy and was

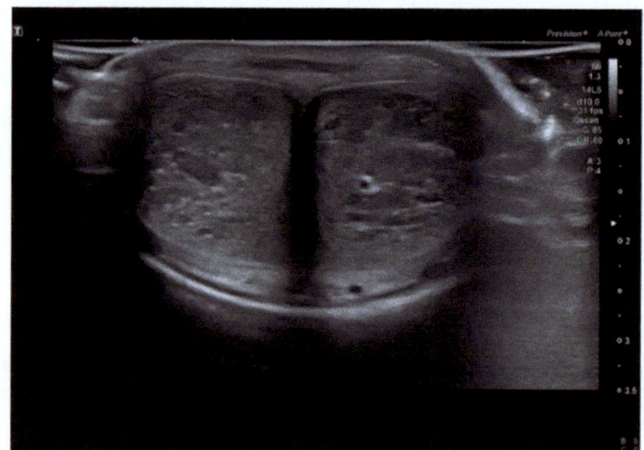

Fig. 17.1 Round and ecogenic cavernous bodies representing hard erection

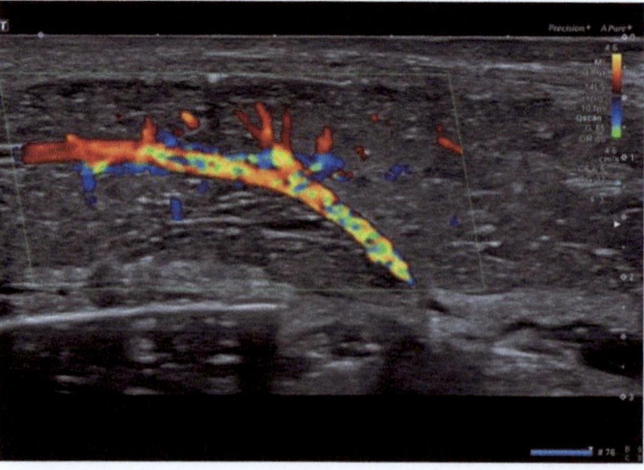

Fig. 17.2 Normal cavernous artery hemodynamic status in color mode with aliasing artifact demontrating high velocities or even assumption of reverse diastole

Fig. 17.3 Spectral Doppler analysiswith high sistolic velocity peak and reverse diatole representing normal hemodynamics

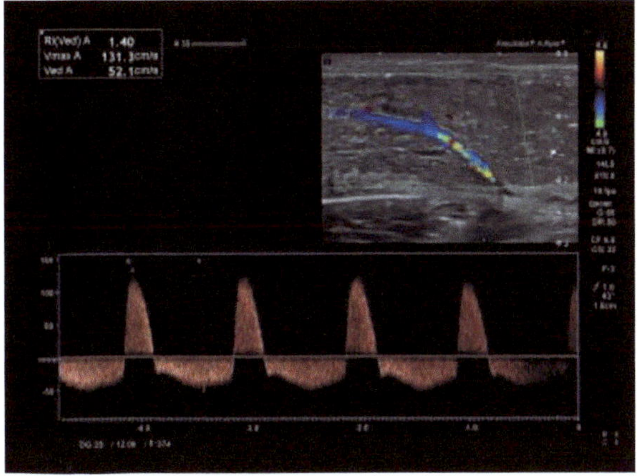

explained that he has a very good prognosis. Note that the patient was administered a relatively low dose of trimix and still needed erection reversal, which is a very important step in PDU studies, especially in cases of psychogenic ED.

17.3   Case 2

A 45-year-old man with no previous medical history or any ongoing use of medication began experiencing pain during erections 2 years ago. After urologic consultation, the patient was prescribed vitamin E, but his symptoms did not improve. A year later, the pain finally disappeared, and the penis presented a dorsal curvature that renders him incapable of performing sexual intercourse, which has made him extremely frustrated. About a month ago, he reported a worsening of the curvature and the onset of erectile dysfunction. During medical interview, it was notable that the patient had a significant decrease on his self-esteem. Upon questioning, the patient reported normal morning hardness and low sexual desire.

The patient was offered a PDU examination for an accurate penile deformity assessment and for a more detailed evaluation of his ED [3, 6], since according to the provided information the patient was very likely to undergo surgical intervention for his penile condition. After injection of 10 units of standard trimix, a rigid erection was obtained (EHS 4 or 10/10) as demonstrated in Fig. 17.4. A complete examination during PDU is demonstrated in Figs. 17.5, 17.6, and 17.7. After 1 h of trimix injection, the patient did not have rigidity sufficient for penetration (EHS 2 or 5/10) and was discharged [4].

Commentary: This is a classical presentation of Peyronie's disease with painful erections associated to acquired penile deformities. In this case, PDU examination is highly indicated to allow for a formal documentation of penile curvature and adequate planning of a surgical approach [3, 6]. Examiners must be certified that maximal rigidity was obtained during the examination as poor erections might

Fig. 17.4 Documentation
of the curvature in full
hardness erection

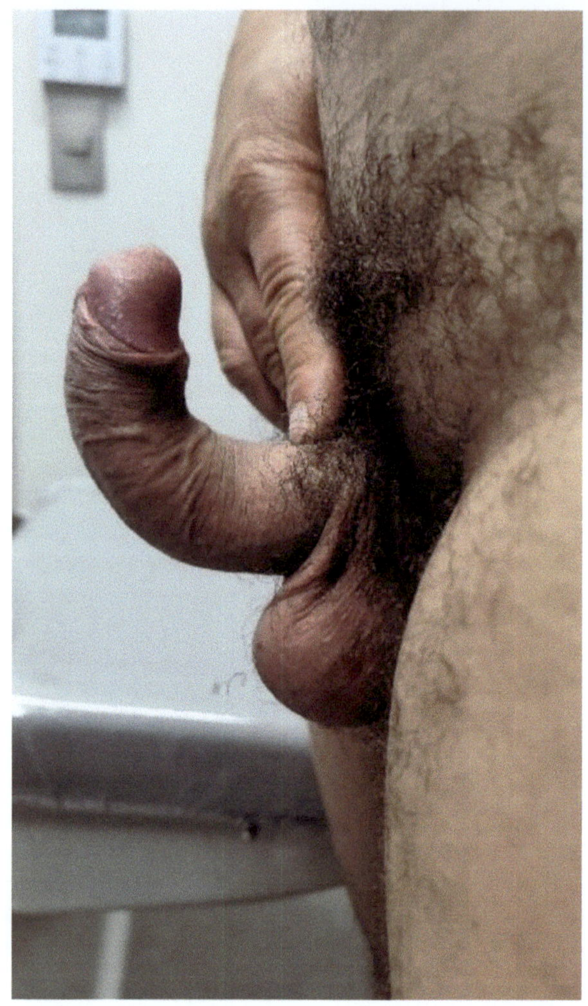

Fig. 17.5 Normal
cavernous artery
hemodynamic in
color mode

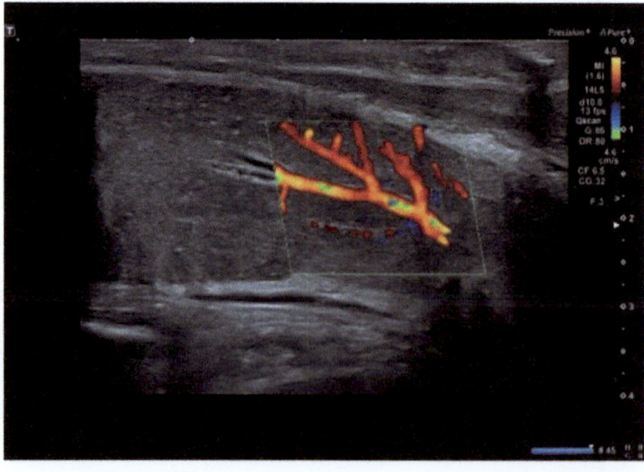

Fig. 17.6 Normal representation of hemodynamic in spectral Doppler mode showing vascular integrity

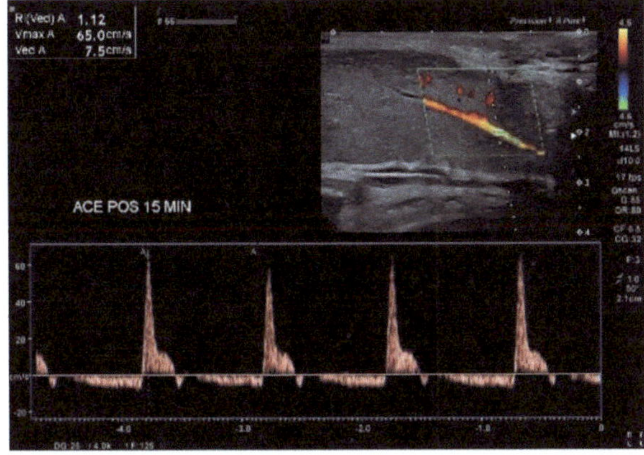

Fig. 17.7 B-mode of a transversal image of the cavernous bodies showing dorsal calcified plaque within the tunica albuginea and intracavernous calcifications

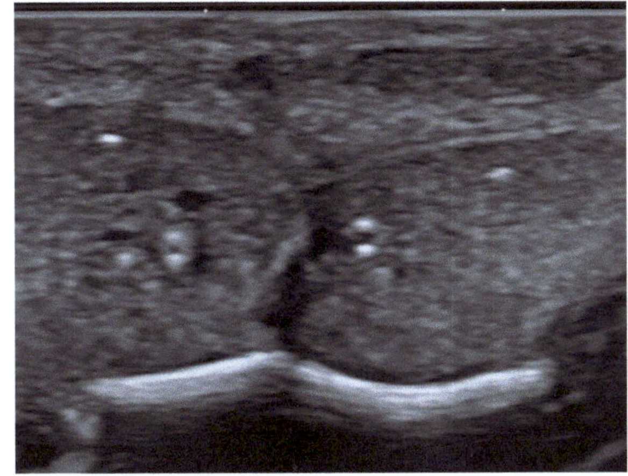

underestimate curvatures or associated penile deformities. It is also important to perform hemodynamic evaluation of the penis in these cases because PDU has proved to be superior to medical history taking or use of validated questionnaires in the assessment of erectile function in patients with Peyronie's disease. Moreover, although there are many possible facets related to the pathophysiology of ED in men with Peyronie's disease, the psychogenic nature is still the most prevalent one [4].

17.4   Case 3

A 72-year-old patient presented complaining of progressive erectile dysfunction for 5 years. Initially, the patient was responsive to oral medication to improve erections, but for the last 2 years, oral treatment lost its efficacy and he was no longer able to engage in penetrative sexual activity. The patient's previous medical history was remarkable for his poorly controlled comorbidities including diabetes, hypercholesterolemia, and hypertension. The patient also mentioned the abolishment of his morning erections. Recently, the patient tried intracavernous injection of alprostadil and did not obtain sufficient rigidity for penetration, and a PDU examination was ordered.

On the exam day, the patient failed to obtain adequate rigidity (EHS 2, 3/10) even after redosing of intracavernous agents in a total of 100 units of trimix [4]. Multiple US readings were performed at different time points, whose findings are demonstrated in Figs. 17.8, 17.9, and 17.10, and the patient received the diagnosis of bilateral arterial insufficiency.

Commentary: This is a classic history of a case with organic ED, possibly related to vasculogenic mechanisms [1, 2]. This elderly patient with multiple comorbidities and poor medical control had long-term history of ED, which had already failed multiple attempts of erectile pharmacotherapy. Despite high doses of vasoactive agents during the exam, his penile hemodynamics could be compensated. This

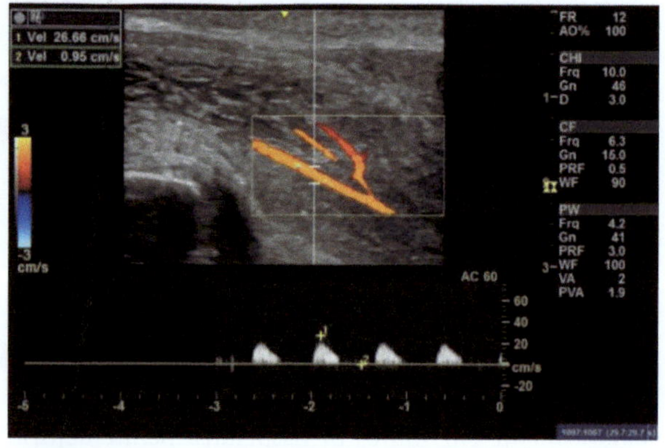

Fig. 17.8 Show low systolic velocity peak insufficient to achieve a hard erection

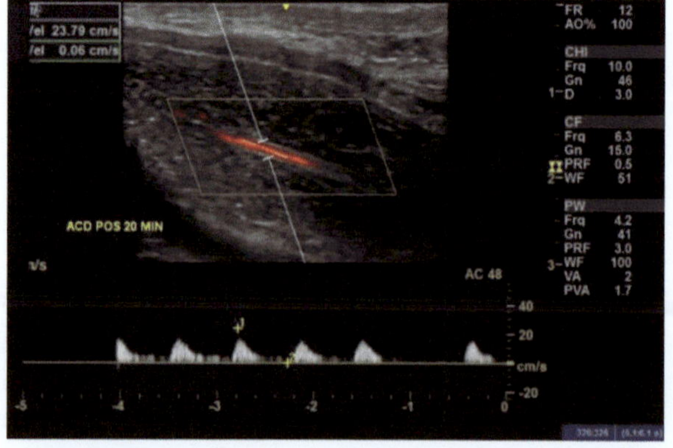

Fig. 17.9 After full dose of trimix, systolic velocity peak is still low and not enough for maintaining a hard erection

Fig. 17.10 Transverse image of the hypoechogenic cavernous body means that they are compressive and not totally filled with blood

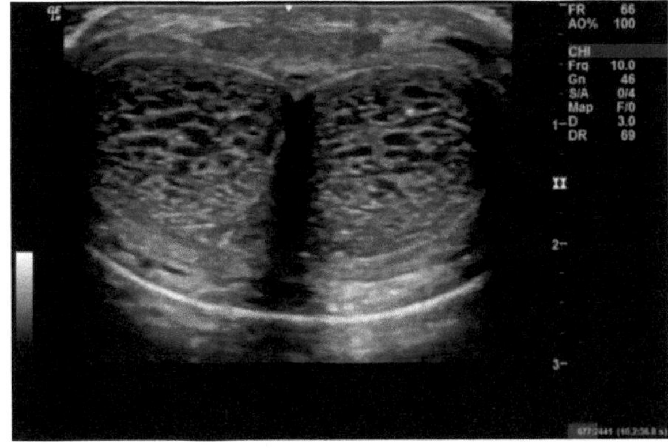

finding usually indicates a poor prognosis, and this patient is likely not going to have enough rigidity for penetration with any noninvasive treatment option available. If a penetrative sex life is still desired, penile implant surgery is the best option and the patient should be counseled accordingly [2, 5].

17.5 Case 4

A 67-year-old patient with no comorbidities presented with erectile dysfunction following radical prostatectomy for a locally advanced prostate cancer 8 months years ago. Prior to surgery, he had a satisfactory erectile function with successful penetration in most of his sexual encounters, but now the patient is irresponsive to PDE5i and has not engaged in penetrative intercourse ever since the operation. The patient was in a health stable relationship and had preserved libido. The patient denied the presence of nocturnal erections but had noticed that his erection would become slightly better in orthostatic position, but enough for penetration. He was counseled to try intracavernous therapy to treat his ED, but the he was afraid of needles and preferred to proceed with PDU at that moment.

During PDU, the patient was able to obtain a 6/10 (EHS 3), which was similar to his best quality erection (BQE) after 82 units of standard trimix [6]. Figures 17.11 and 17.12 demonstrated US findings during peak rigidity. These findings were consistent with cavernous veno-occlusive dysfunction, with high PSVs (>30 cm/s) and high EDVs (>5 cm/s) despite high dosage of trimix. The patient started to refer a diffuse penile pain at the end of PDU, most likely related to the injection of alprostadil in the regimen of intracavernous agents.

Commentary: The patient in case 4 is one of the most common examples of a dysfunctional veno-occlusive mechanism. He had previous history of radical prostatectomy, which is a known risk factor for the development of smooth muscle collagenization. Having better erections in the standing position is an indicative of gravitational changes of penile rigidity, which is most often seen in veno-occlusive

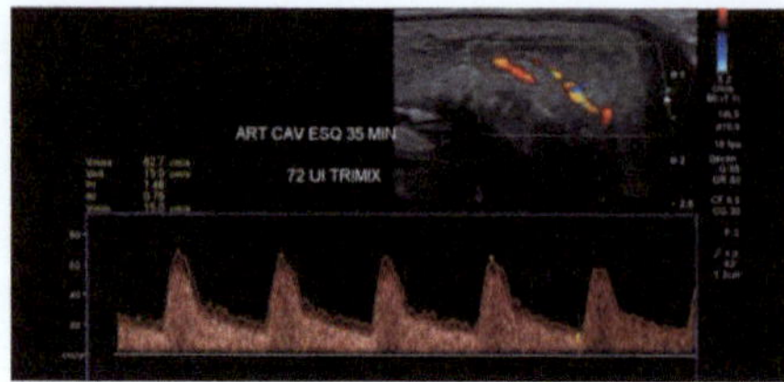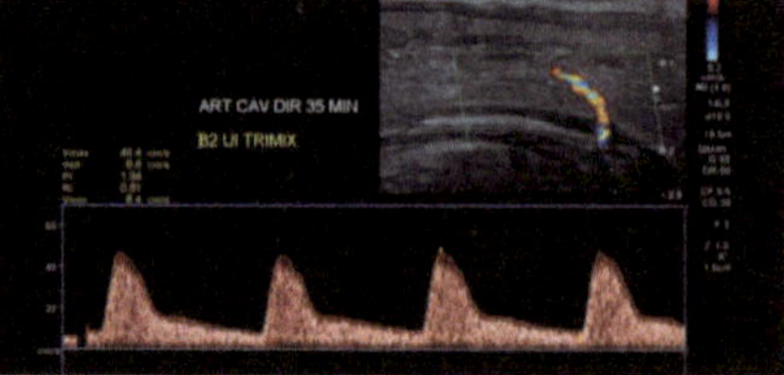

Fig. 17.11 Even with high doses of trimix, still very high ending diastolic velocities are found, indicating venous leak

Fig. 17.12 Transversal image of hypoechogenic compressive cavernous body representing penile sinusoids not fully complete

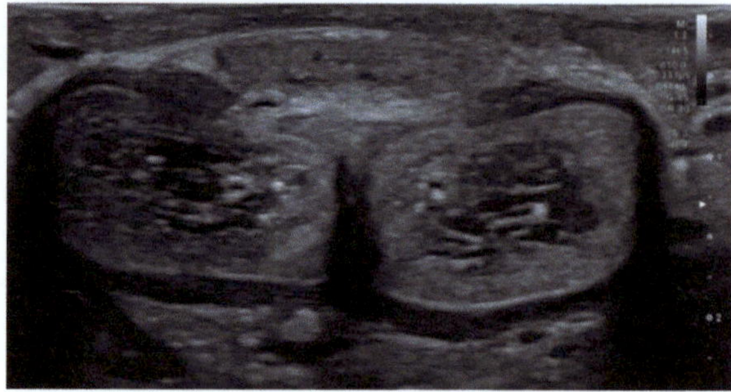

dysfunction [4]. The most common differential diagnosis would be high-grade psychogenic ED, which did not seem to be the case as the patient was adequately redosed with trimix and did not seem overtly anxious at the time of PDU. Although it has been reported that patients may improve their erectile function after radical prostatectomy up to 2 years after surgery as a result of nerve recovery, in this case the patient has already developed smooth muscle degeneration. Therefore, this condition is likely not going to improve over time, and definitive treatment options such as immediate penile implant would be an interesting treatment option.

17.6 Conclusions

This chapter offers a valuable collection of case studies that demonstrate the clinical application and diagnostic value of penile Doppler ultrasound in the evaluation of male sexual health. By presenting real-world scenarios, it provides readers with practical insights into the use of this imaging technique and its impact on patient management. This chapter serves as a valuable resource for clinicians, sonographers, and researchers involved in penile Doppler ultrasound and its role in the comprehensive assessment of penile vascular disorders.

References

1. Salonia A, Bettocchi C, Boeri L, Capogrosso P, Carvalho J, Cilesiz NC, et al. European Association of Urology guidelines on sexual and reproductive health-2021 update: male sexual dysfunction. Eur Urol. 2021;80(3):333–57.
2. Yafi FA, Jenkins L, Albersen M, Corona G, Isidori AM, Goldfarb S, et al. Erectile dysfunction. Nat Rev Dis Primers. 2016;2:16003.
3. Sikka SC, Hellstrom WJ, Brock G, Morales AM. Standardization of vascular assessment of erectile dysfunction: standard operating procedures for duplex ultrasound. J Sex Med. 2013;10(1):120–9.
4. Nascimento B, Miranda EP, Terrier JE, Carneiro F, Mulhall JP. A critical analysis of methodology pitfalls in duplex Doppler ultrasound in the evaluation of patients with erectile dysfunction: technical and interpretation deficiencies. J Sex Med. 2020;17(8):1416–22.
5. Ma M, Yu B, Qin F, Yuan J. Current approaches to the diagnosis of vascular erectile dysfunction. Transl Androl Urol. 2020;9(2):709.
6. Carneiro F, Saito OC, Miranda EP. Standardization of penile hemodynamic evaluation through color duplex-doppler ultrasound. Rev Assoc Méd Bras. 2020;66:1180–6.

Index

© The Editor(s) (if applicable) and The Author(s), under exclusive license to Springer Nature Switzerland AG 2024
E. d. P. Miranda, F. Carneiro, *Penile Color Duplex-Doppler Ultrasound in Erectile Dysfunction Diagnosis and Management*,
https://doi.org/10.1007/978-3-031-55649-4

MIX
Papier aus verantwortungsvollen Quellen
Paper from responsible sources
FSC® C105338

If you have any concerns about our products,
you can contact us on
ProductSafety@springernature.com

In case Publisher is established outside the EU,
the EU authorized representative is:
**Springer Nature Customer Service Center GmbH
Europaplatz 3, 69115 Heidelberg, Germany**

Printed by Libri Plureos GmbH
in Hamburg, Germany